Guide to
Calories

Guide to Calories

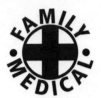

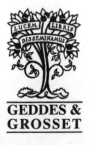

**GEDDES &
GROSSET**

Published by Geddes & Grosset,
David Dale House, New Lanark, ML11 9DJ, Scotland

© 2005 Geddes & Grosset

Published 2005

ISBN 1 84205 539 9

Printed and bound in Poland

POLSKABOOK

Contents

Introduction

Why are people overweight? The simple answer is that they overeat. This means that more energy (calories) is taken in through food than is expended (activity). This simple truth can be expressed in the form of the 'Energy Equation':

Calories *in, more than* Energy *out* = Weight *gain*

The excess calories are stored as body fat and excess weight is the result.

Whatever you might think, having 'big bones' or a 'heavy frame' do not necessarily make you fat.

In practical terms, you must alter the energy equation so that your calorie input is less than your activity output. You can do this simply by reducing the amount you eat.

For *safe and healthy* weight loss, do not reduce your total daily calories below 1000 unless you are under medical supervision. When you drastically cut your food intake, your body perceives a state of starvation and adjusts the metabolic rate to cope on the reduced amount of 'fuel'. This means that you will not lose weight. If you then increase your food intake, your body's lowered metabolic rate does not burn it up so effectively, so you will gain even more weight.

Don't get caught in this irritating 'Catch 22'. Reduce calorie intake gradually and you will achieve a steady and more lasting reduction in weight.

For *most effective* weight loss, increase your daily activity as well as reducing your calories (*see* Exercise, page 98).

Counting Calories

Slimming seems simple, yet many slimmers fail because our relationship with food is a complex one. Successful slimming is based upon knowledge of the following:

- psychological factors that affect efforts to diet
- appropriate action

Things you should know about

Weighing yourself

This does not have to be a depressing or self-deceiving exercise if you keep to a few rules:

- **Use** the same scales.
- **Keep** the scales in *exactly* the same place or they may weigh differently.
- **Weigh** at the same time of the day, preferably first thing in the morning.
- **Wear** a similar weight of clothes, preferably none.
- **Weigh** yourself only once a week. Weight loss is a relatively slow process, so don't court disappointment by weighing yourself more often. Too frequent weighing may also encourage obsession.
- **Stand** still on the scales, distributing your weight evenly.
- Advertisements – and other people – sometimes boast of weight losses that are both huge and fast, and may create unrealistic expectations in you.
- Try not to be impatient. Weight lost rapidly may be unhealthy and may be regained equally rapidly.
- As a rough guide, a safe and healthy weight loss for most people is an *average* of 1 kg/2 lb per week. Note that weight loss may vary from week to week.

Weight loss and contraception

Women using the diaphragm method of birth control should note that a weight loss of more than 3 kg/7 lb could mean that their contraceptive device no longer fits properly and that pregnancy might result. Remember to consult your family planning adviser as soon as necessary.

PMS and slimming

Woman who suffer from PMS (Pre-menstrual Syndrome), sometimes find that, for a few days before a period, temporary fluid retention causes additional weight and may mask an actual fat loss.

Other symptoms of PMS, such as depression, tension or a craving for carbohydrates, may also adversely affect dieting behaviour. Keep notes of your symptoms and consult your doctor and/or one of the national associations concerned with PMS (*see* Useful Addresses and Further Reading).

'Change of Life'

Menopausal symptoms may cause problems that also interfere with your slimming efforts. Do not feel that you are doomed to suffer unaided. You could consult your doctor, a well-woman clinic, and/or the books suggested (*see* Useful Addresses and Further Reading). If your doctor proves unsympathetic, remember that you are entitled to change your GP if you wish.

Eating with the family

Slimmers can easily eat with the family if they follow the guidelines in Cook Slim. Delicious meals can be created, which will have health benefits for the whole family. Families can be very resistant to change, so make changes to the family meals without drawing attention to them.

Entertaining

Apply the Cook Slim guidelines here too. Your dinner guests will never suspect – they will merely be delighted with the results!

Look out for cookery books containing low-fat recipes (*see* Useful Reading) and amend your favourite recipes as the Cook Slim guidelines suggest.

Your Ideal Weight

It is important to remember that height/weight charts supply only a general guide to suitable weights. They are often based upon statistics from life insurance companies and show desirable, 'healthy' weights in relation to height. However, individuals vary greatly and what might be ideal for one person's frame may not be so for another. Consequently, most height/weight charts provide a range of acceptable weights relative to each height.

Using the chart

- **Do** get some help to check your height – don't guess.
- **Do not** set yourself an ideal weight so far below your existing weight that it intimidates you immediately. It is not always necessary to set a target at the outset. You could simply allow yourself to lose some weight and thus gain confidence first.
- **Do** use common sense in assessing your shape and the amount of obvious body fat. However, it is not always easy to see yourself objectively, so also ask the opinion of someone you trust and/or your doctor.
- **Do** remember that it is natural for women to have more body fat than men.
- **Do not** become obsessed about your weight or shape. You *do not* have to match some fashion magazine ideal.

Calorie intake requirements

The calorie intake needs of the average human body are dependent upon age and level of activity. Children require a greater energy input for their weight compared to adults.

Counting Calories

A calorie or kilocalorie (kcal) is a unit of energy. This is the measure of the exact amount of heat required to increase the temperature of 1000 g of water by 1° C. The term kilojoule (kJ) is often used. 1 kcal = 4.2 kJ.

Determining the need to diet

It is only necessary to diet to safeguard your health if your weight is sufficiently great to put you at risk of developing the disorders of obesity such as high blood pressure, heart and circulatory disease and diabetes.

Body mass index (BMI)

In order to determine when this point is reached, scientists and doctors use a formula known as the body mass index, or BMI, which is calculated from measurements of height and weight. A scale of numbers is derived, ranging from 'morbidly obese' at the top to 'emaciated' at the bottom and each person is classified according to his or her individual reading. The BMI figure is arrived at by using the following calculation:

weight (in kilograms) ÷ height (in metres) squared i.e.

$$\frac{\text{weight in kg}}{\text{height in m}^2}$$

To derive your height in metres, calculate your height in inches and divide the number by 40, i.e.:

$$\frac{\text{height in inches}}{40}$$

To derive your weight in kilograms, calculate your weight in pounds and divide the number by 2.2, i.e.:

$$\frac{\text{weight in pounds}}{2.2}$$

Example:

A woman 5 ft 4 in tall is 64/40 in = 1.6 metres high and weighing 9 stone 7 lbs (133lbs) is 133/2.2 = 60.45 kg.

Table 1: BMI Imperial Measurements

Your height in inches

Weight in pounds	58	59	60	61	62	63	64	65	66	67	68	69	70	71	72
90	19	18	18	17	17	16	15	15	15	14	14	13	13	13	12
92	19	19	18	17	17	16	16	15	15	14	14	14	13	13	13
94	20	19	18	18	17	17	16	16	15	15	14	14	14	13	13
96	20	19	19	18	18	17	17	16	16	15	15	14	14	13	13
98	21	20	19	19	18	17	17	16	16	15	15	15	14	14	13
100	21	20	20	19	18	18	17	17	16	16	15	15	14	14	14
102	21	21	20	19	19	18	18	17	17	16	16	15	15	14	14
104	22	21	20	20	19	18	18	17	17	16	16	15	15	14	14
106	22	21	21	20	19	19	18	18	17	17	16	16	15	15	14
108	23	22	21	20	20	19	18	18	17	17	16	16	15	15	15
110	23	22	22	21	20	20	19	18	18	17	17	16	15	15	15
112	23	23	22	21	21	20	19	19	18	18	17	17	16	16	15
114	24	23	22	22	21	20	20	19	18	18	17	17	16	16	16
116	24	23	22	22	21	21	20	19	19	18	17	17	16	16	16
118	25	24	23	22	22	21	20	20	19	19	18	17	17	17	16
120	25	24	24	23	22	21	21	20	19	19	18	18	17	17	16

Counting Calories

Weight in pounds	\ Your height in inches 58	59	60	61	62	63	64	65	66	67	68	69	70	71	72
122	26	25	24	23	22	22	21	20	20	19	19	18	18	17	17
124	26	25	24	23	23	22	21	21	20	19	19	18	18	17	17
126	26	26	25	24	23	22	22	21	20	20	19	19	18	18	17
128	27	26	25	24	23	23	22	21	21	20	20	19	18	18	17
130	27	26	25	25	24	23	22	22	21	20	20	19	19	18	18
132	28	27	26	25	24	23	23	22	21	21	20	20	19	18	18
134	28	27	26	25	25	24	23	22	22	21	20	20	19	19	18
136	29	28	27	26	25	24	24	23	22	21	21	20	20	19	18
138	29	28	27	26	25	25	24	23	22	22	21	20	20	19	19
140	29	28	27	27	26	25	24	23	23	22	21	21	20	20	19
142	30	29	28	27	26	26	25	24	23	22	22	21	20	20	20
144	30	29	28	27	26	26	25	24	23	23	22	21	21	20	20
146	31	30	29	28	27	26	25	25	24	23	22	22	21	20	20
148	31	30	29	28	27	27	26	25	24	23	23	22	21	21	20
150	31	30	29	28	28	27	26	25	26	24	23	22	22	21	20
152	32	31	30	29	28	27	26	26	26	24	23	23	22	21	21
154	32	31	30	29	28	27	27	26	25	24	23	23	22	22	21

Your height in inches

Weight in pounds

Weight (lbs)	58	59	60	61	62	63	64	65	66	67	68	69	70	71	72
156	33	32	31	30	29	28	27	26	25	24	24	23	22	22	21
158	33	32	31	30	29	28	27	26	26	25	24	23	23	22	21
160	34	32	31	30	29	28	27	27	26	25	24	24	23	22	22
162	34	33	32	31	30	29	28	27	26	25	25	24	23	23	22
164	34	33	32	31	30	29	28	27	26	26	25	24	24	23	22
166	35	34	32	31	30	29	28	28	27	26	25	25	24	23	23
168	35	34	33	32	31	30	29	28	27	26	26	25	24	23	23
170	36	34	33	32	31	30	29	28	27	27	26	25	24	24	23
172	36	35	34	32	31	30	30	29	28	27	26	25	25	24	23
174	36	35	34	33	32	31	30	29	28	27	26	26	25	24	24
176	37	36	34	33	32	31	30	29	28	28	27	26	25	25	24
178	37	36	35	34	33	32	31	30	29	28	27	26	26	25	24
180	38	36	35	34	33	32	31	30	29	28	27	27	26	25	24
182	38	37	36	34	33	32	31	30	29	29	28	27	26	25	25
184	39	37	36	35	34	33	32	31	30	29	28	27	26	26	25
186	39	38	36	35	34	33	32	31	30	29	28	27	27	26	25
188	39	38	37	36	34	33	32	31	30	29	29	28	27	26	26

Counting Calories

Your height in inches

Weight in pounds

Weight in pounds	58	59	60	61	62	63	64	65	66	67	68	69	70	71	72
190	40	38	37	36	35	34	33	32	31	30	29	28	27	27	26
192	40	39	38	36	35	34	33	32	31	30	29	28	28	27	26
194	41	39	38	37	36	34	33	32	31	30	30	29	28	27	26
196	41	40	38	37	36	35	34	33	32	31	30	29	28	27	27
198	41	40	39	38	36	35	34	33	32	31	30	29	28	28	27
200	42	41	39	38	37	36	34	33	32	31	30	30	29	28	27
202	42	41	40	38	37	36	35	34	33	32	31	30	29	28	27
204	43	41	40	39	37	36	35	34	33	32	31	30	29	29	28
206	43	42	40	39	38	37	35	34	33	32	32	31	30	29	28
208	44	42	41	39	38	37	36	35	34	33	32	31	30	29	28
210	44	43	41	40	39	37	36	35	34	33	32	31	30	29	29
212	44	43	42	40	39	38	36	35	34	33	32	31	31	30	29
214	45	43	42	41	39	38	37	36	34	34	33	32	31	30	29
216	45	44	42	41	40	39	37	36	35	34	33	32	31	30	29
218	46	44	43	41	40	39	38	36	35	34	33	32	31	30	30
220	46	45	43	42	40	39	38	37	36	35	34	33	32	31	30

Table 2: BMI Metric Measurements

Your height in centimetres

Weight in kg

	150	152.5	155	157.5	160	162.5	165	167.5	170	172.5	175	177.5	180	182.5	185	187.5	190
40	18	17	17	16	16	15	15	14	14	13	13	13	12	12	12	11	11
41	18	18	17	17	16	16	15	15	14	14	13	13	13	12	12	11	11
42	19	18	17	17	16	16	15	15	15	14	14	13	13	13	12	12	12
43	19	18	18	17	17	16	16	15	15	14	14	13	13	13	13	12	12
44	20	19	18	18	17	17	16	16	15	15	14	14	14	13	13	13	12
45	20	19	19	18	18	17	17	16	16	15	15	14	14	14	13	13	12
46	20	20	19	19	18	17	17	16	16	15	15	15	14	14	13	13	13
47	21	20	20	19	18	18	17	17	16	16	15	15	15	14	14	13	13
48	21	21	20	19	19	18	18	17	17	16	16	15	15	14	14	14	13
49	22	21	20	20	19	19	18	17	17	16	16	16	15	15	14	14	14
50	22	22	21	20	20	19	18	18	17	17	16	16	15	15	15	14	14
51	23	22	21	21	20	19	19	18	18	17	17	16	16	16	15	15	14
52	23	22	22	21	20	20	19	19	18	17	17	17	16	16	15	15	14
53	24	23	22	21	21	20	19	19	18	18	17	17	16	16	16	15	15
54	24	23	23	22	21	20	20	19	19	18	18	17	17	16	16	15	15
55	24	24	23	22	21	21	20	20	19	18	18	17	17	17	16	16	15
56	25	24	23	23	22	21	21	20	19	19	18	18	17	17	16	16	16

Counting Calories

Your height in centimetres

Weight in kg

Weight (kg)	150	152.5	155	157.5	160	162.5	165	167.5	170	172.5	175	177.5	180	182.5	185	187.5	190
57	25	25	24	23	22	22	21	20	20	19	19	18	18	17	17	16	16
58	26	25	24	23	23	22	21	21	20	19	19	18	18	17	17	16	16
59	26	25	25	24	23	22	22	21	20	20	19	19	18	18	17	17	16
60	27	26	25	24	23	23	22	21	21	20	20	19	19	18	18	17	17
61	27	26	25	25	24	23	22	22	21	20	20	19	19	18	18	17	17
62	28	27	26	25	24	23	23	22	21	21	20	20	19	19	18	18	17
63	28	27	26	25	25	24	23	22	22	21	21	20	19	19	18	18	17
64	28	28	27	26	25	24	24	23	22	22	21	20	20	19	19	18	18
65	29	28	27	26	25	25	24	23	22	22	21	21	20	19	19	18	18
66	29	28	27	27	26	25	24	24	23	22	22	21	20	20	19	19	18
67	30	29	28	27	26	25	25	24	23	23	22	21	21	20	20	19	18
68	30	29	28	27	27	26	25	24	24	23	22	22	21	20	20	19	19
69	31	30	29	28	27	26	26	25	24	23	23	22	21	20	20	20	19
70	31	30	29	28	27	27	26	25	24	24	23	22	22	21	20	20	19
71	32	31	30	29	28	27	26	25	25	24	23	23	22	21	21	20	19
72	32	31	30	29	28	27	27	26	25	24	24	23	22	21	21	21	20
73	32	31	30	29	29	28	27	26	25	25	24	23	23	22	21	21	20
74	33	32	31	30	29	28	28	26	26	25	24	23	23	22	22	21	20
75	33	32	31	30	29	28	28	27	26	25	24	24	23	23	22	21	21

Your height in centimetres

Weight in kg

	150	152.5	155	157.5	160	162.5	165	167.5	170	172.5	175	177.5	180	182.5	185	187.5	190
76	34	33	32	31	30	29	28	27	26	25	24	23	23	23	22	22	21
77	34	33	32	31	30	29	28	27	27	26	25	24	24	23	22	22	21
78	35	34	32	31	30	30	29	28	27	26	25	25	24	23	23	22	22
79	35	34	33	32	31	30	29	28	27	27	26	25	24	24	23	22	22
80	36	34	33	32	31	30	29	29	28	27	26	25	25	24	23	23	22
81	36	35	34	33	32	31	30	29	28	27	26	26	25	24	24	23	22
82	36	35	34	33	32	31	30	29	28	28	27	26	25	25	24	23	23
83	37	36	35	33	32	31	30	30	29	28	27	26	26	25	24	24	23
84	37	36	35	34	33	32	31	30	29	28	27	27	26	25	24	24	23
85	38	37	35	34	33	32	31	30	29	29	28	27	26	26	25	24	24
86	38	37	36	35	34	33	32	31	30	29	28	27	27	26	25	24	24
87	39	37	36	35	34	33	32	31	30	29	28	28	27	26	25	25	24
88	39	38	37	35	34	33	32	31	30	30	29	28	27	26	26	25	24
89	40	38	37	36	35	34	33	32	31	30	29	28	27	27	26	25	25
90	40	39	37	36	35	34	33	32	31	30	29	29	28	27	26	26	25
91	40	39	38	37	36	34	33	32	31	31	30	29	28	27	26	26	25
92	41	40	38	37	36	35	34	33	32	31	30	29	28	28	27	26	25
93	41	40	39	37	36	35	34	33	32	31	30	30	29	28	27	26	26
94	42	40	39	38	37	36	35	34	33	32	31	30	29	28	27	27	26

Counting Calories

Your height in centimetres

Weight in kg

	150	152.5	155	157.5	160	162.5	165	167.5	170	172.5	175	177.5	180	182.5	185	187.5	190
95	42	41	40	39	37	36	35	34	33	32	31	30	29	29	28	27	26
96	43	41	40	39	38	36	35	34	33	32	31	30	30	29	28	27	27
97	43	42	40	39	38	37	36	35	34	33	32	31	30	29	28	28	27
98	44	42	41	40	38	37	36	35	34	33	32	31	30	29	29	28	27
99	44	43	41	40	39	37	36	35	34	33	32	31	31	30	29	28	27
100	44	43	42	40	39	38	37	36	35	34	33	32	31	30	29	29	28

Hence her BMI is:

$$\frac{60.45 \text{ kg}}{1.6\text{m}^2} = \frac{60.45}{1.6 \times 1.6} = \frac{60.45}{2.56} = 23.6$$

Since these calculations are quite complex BMIs for both metric and Imperial measurements are given in tables 1 and 2 on pages 13 to 20. Find your height and weight on one of the charts to discover your round BMI figure.

The BMI scale is classified as follows:

Less than 15   Emaciated
15 to 19   Underweight
19 to 25   Average
25 to 27   Overweight
27 to 30   Overweight and at risk of developing obesity related diseases
30 to 40   Obese and at high risk of disease
40 +   Morbidly obese

Designation of the optimum BMI range, associated with the lowest risk of weight-related conditions and illnesses, varies somewhat between different countries. However, in general terms, an optimum BMI for adults lies within the range of 20 to 25. For women it is in the order of 18.8 to 23.4 and for men, 19.8 to 24. Anyone lying slightly above or slightly below these figures is not at risk but still might wish to keep an eye on their weight. In fact using the example given above of a woman 5 ft 4 in tall; with an optimum BMI range of 20 to 25, her weight could be anything from 8 st 4 lbs (52.7 kg) to 10 st 8 lbs. (67 kg). In order to reach the danger zone of a BMI of 27, when she would be at risk of developing obesity-related diseases, her weight would need to climb to 11 st 3 lbs (71.3 kg) or above.

However, it is probable that at this weight, or even some way below it, many women would feel that they would like to lose a few pounds! Conversely, women especially, are at some risk if their BMI is too low and anyone with a figure of 19 or below should make sure that they are eating a full, healthy, well-balanced diet.

No one with a BMI of less than 20 should go on a diet – with this reading, you *cannot* be overweight. Equally, if your BMI is 30 or above, seek medical advice about losing weight rather than embarking upon a diet on your own.

BMI is the most reliable measurement for determining health risks associated with weight but, as has been seen, it allows for considerable variation. Other figures that are used, especially by diet books and the diet industry in general, are so-called 'standard', 'average' or 'ideal' weight for height charts for men and women. These can be extremely variable, depending upon which book you are reading and should only be used as a rough guide. It is, after all, in the interests of the diet industry to promote ideal weights on the lower scale in order to recruit potential dieters!

Weight charts are often based on ideal or standard weights for young adults and fail to take into account that people naturally tend to get a little heavier in middle and older age. Health experts advise people to try to retain the weight and clothes size that they had in youth (as long as they were not overweight). However, it may be more realistic to try and remain within sight of that weight and to keep muscles well-toned by taking plenty of exercise!

Frame size

The most useful weight charts are those which take into account body frame size, i.e. the mass of the internal skeleton.

Table 3: Medium frame determined by elbow width

WOMEN		MEN	
Height in m and feet	Elbow width in cm and ins	Height in m and feet	Elbow width in cm and ins
1.45 to 1.47 m (4' 9" to 4' 10")	5.7 cm (2" to 2+")	1.55 to 1.60 m (5' 1" to 5' 3")	6.4 to 7 cm (2+" to 2+")
1.50 to 1.57 m (4' 11" to 5' 2")	5.4 to 6.4 cm (2" to 2+")	1.63 to 1.68 m (5' 4" to 5' 6")	6.7 to 7.3 cm (2" to 2")
1.60 to 1.68 m (5' 3" to 5' 6")	5.7 to 6.7 cm (2+" to 2")	1.70 to 1.78 m (5' 7" to 5' 10")	7 to 7.6 cm (2+" to 3")
1.70 to 1.78 m (5' 7" to 5' 10")	6 to 7 cm (2" to 2+")	1.80 to 1.88 m (5'11" to 6' 2")	7.3 to 7.9 cm (2" to 3")
1.80 to 1.85 m (5'11" to 6'1")	6.4 to 7.3 cm (2+" to 3")	1.90 to 1.93 m (6' 3" to 6' 4")	7.6 to 8.3 cm (3" to 3+")

In general, women have a smaller body frame than men (although there is inevitably some overlap between the two) but people of the same sex and height also vary considerably in bone structure. A common excuse among those who are somewhat overweight is to assert that it is because they have 'large bones' but, in fact, the skeleton is relatively light compared to soft tissue!

A large-framed person can expect to weigh more than one with a smaller frame and can more readily accommodate extra weight without appearing to be fat. Frame size can be estimated by measuring the width of the arm at the elbow. In order to do this, you should place a piece of paper on a table and then kneel or sit facing it and place your upper arm on the paper. The upper arm should be flat on the paper with the forearm in the air at an angle of 90° at the

Table 4: Tables for standard body weight
MEN

Height ft (m)	Small Frame lbs (kg)	Medium Frame lbs (kg)	Large Frame lbs (kg)
5' 1" (1.55)	107–130 (49–59)	113–134 (51–61)	121–140 (55–64)
5' 2" (1.57)	110–132 (50–60)	116–138 (53–63)	124–144 (56–65)
5' 3" (1.60)	113–134 (51–61)	119–140 (54–64)	127–150 (58–68)
5' 4" (1.63)	116–135 (53–61)	122–142 (55–65)	131–154 (59–70)
5' 5" (1.65)	119–137 (54–62)	125–146 (57–66)	133–159 (60–72)
5' 6" (1.68)	123–140 (56–64)	129–149 (59–68)	137–163 (62–74)
5' 7" (1.70)	127–143 (58–65)	133–152 (60–69)	142–167 (64–76)
5' 8" (1.73)	131–145 (60–66)	137–155 (62–71)	146–171 (66–78)
5' 9" (1.75)	135–149 (61–68)	141–158 (64–72)	150–175 (68–80)
5' 10" (1.78)	139–152 (63–69)	145–161 (66–73)	154–179 (70–81)
5' 11" (1.80)	143–155 (65–70)	149–165 (68–75)	159–183 (72–83)
6' (1.83)	147–159 (67–72)	153–169 (70–77)	163–187 (74–85)
6' 1" (1.85)	151–165 (69–75)	157–175 (71–80)	167–189 (76–86)
6' 2" (1.88)	155–168 (70–76)	161–179 (73–81)	171–197 (78–89)
6' 3" (1.90)	157–173 (72–79)	166–185 (75–84)	176–202 (80–92)

elbow. Using the thumb and index finger of the other hand, find the bones on either side of the elbow at their widest point. Lower your fingers to the paper, making sure that you maintain the same distance between them and remove your arm. Then, with a pencil, mark the two points on the paper on the inside of your finger and thumb and measure the distance between them, preferably in centimetres. Although not entirely accurate, the measurement gives a reasonable indication of frame size.

Table 3 on page 23 gives the measurements of elbow width for women and men of medium frame at different heights. A larger measurement indicates a large frame and a smaller measurement, a small frame.

WOMEN

Height ft (m)	Small Frame lbs (kg)	Medium Frame lbs (kg)	Large Frame lbs (kg)
4' 10" (1.47)	91–108 (41–49)	95–115 (43–52)	103–119 (47–54)
4' 11" (1.50)	93–112 (42–51)	98–121 (44–55)	106–125 (48–57)
5' (1.52)	96–115 (44–52)	101–124 (46–57)	109–128 (49–58)
5' 1" (1.55)	99–118 (45–54)	104–127 (47–58)	112–131 (51–59)
5' 2" (1.57)	102–121 (46–55)	107–132 (49–60)	115–135 (52–61)
5' 3" (1.60)	105–124 (48–56)	110–135 (50–62)	118–138 (54–63)
5' 4" (1.63)	108–127 (49–58)	113–138 (51–63)	122–142 (55–65)
5' 5" (1.65)	111–130 (50–59)	117–141 (53–64)	126–145 (57–66)
5' 6" (1.68)	115–133 (52–60)	121–144 (55–66)	130–148 (59–67)
5' 7" (1.70)	119–136 (54–62)	125–147 (57–67)	134–151 (61–69)
5' 8" (1.73)	123–139 (56–63)	128–150 (58–68)	137–155 (62–71)
5' 9" (1.75)	127–142 (58–64)	133–153 (60–69)	141–159 (64–73)
5' 10" (1.78)	131–145 (59–66)	137–156 (62–71)	146–165 (66–75)
5' 11" (1.80)	135–148 (61–68)	141–159 (64–72)	150–170 (68–77)
6' (1.83)	138–151 (63–69)	143–163 (65–74)	153–173 (69–79)

Having ascertained your frame size, table 4 on pages 24 to 25, showing a reasonable weight range for people of different heights, can be used as a *guide*. The weights shown are those that are considered to be a standard range for young adults. As previously noted, middle-aged and older people tend to be heavier. Also, people who are athletes, those who carry out weight training or who play a lot of sport and so have developed a great deal of muscle, are heavier simply because muscle weighs more than fat! These factors emphasize the need to interpret the tables sensibly. You may be a little overweight according to the tables, but as long as your BMI lies within the healthy range, there is no medical reason for you to embark upon a diet.

Body shape

Finally, there is one other factor that can be taken in to account when deciding whether you need to lose weight and that is your body shape. There are two main types of body shape – apple and pear – and the category in which you belong is determined by your waist to hip ratio. Use a tape measure to obtain the figures, either in inches or centimetres, and divide the waist measurement by that of the hip. If the number obtained is less than 0.85 for women or 0.95 for men, then you are pear-shaped. If it is more, then you are apple-shaped. Apple-shaped people tend to store excess fat above the waist in their abdomen and this is the more usual pattern for men. Unfortunately, it is associated with a higher risk of the development of obesity-associated diseases and conditions such as heart and circulatory disease, high blood pressure, diabetes and elevated levels of blood cholesterol. The fact that more men than women have this body shape may be one of the reasons why men in western countries are susceptible to heart disease. However, once again, providing that your BMI lies within the healthy range there is no need to do more than endeavour to eat a good low fat diet and take regular exercise. Encouragingly, excess fat above the waist is fairly easy to lose and this is one of the reasons why men who diet are often quite successful.

Pear-shaped people store fat below the waist, around the hips and bottom and in the upper legs. In women, the fat stores here are utilised during pregnancy and breast-feeding and are part of the body's natural resources. For this reason, pear-shaped women often find it difficult to lose fat from these areas. When they go on a diet, they can discover (frustratingly!) that weight is lost above the waist, such as from the bust, where they may already be quite trim, before it starts to come off the desired areas of the hips and thighs. Pear-shaped people are also not immune to heart and circulatory disease and other conditions related to obesity. Hence, like the 'apples', it is sensible for 'pears' to eat a healthy, low-fat diet, incorporate as much exercise as possible into the daily routine and lose weight if BMI or other factors indicate that it is necessary to do so.

Blood cholesterol

Other factors which would indicate that a change of diet is necessary is a high level of blood cholesterol, as this is certainly a risk factor in the development of atheroma and atherosclerosis (furring of the arteries). A high level of blood cholesterol is related to the consumption of a western diet rich in saturated fats, with those who are overweight or obese known to be vulnerable. However, the relationship with body weight is not necessarily a simple, straightforward one and it is possible for people who are not particularly overweight to have elevated blood cholesterol levels. The most accurate way to ascertain your level of cholesterol is by analysis of a blood sample, (although there are some 'over the counter' kits available from chemists and pharmacists). Most medical centres now run Well Woman and Well Man Clinics and a check on blood cholesterol levels is one of the preventative health care measures that is offered to patients. A regular health checkup is advisable for all middle-aged and older people but anyone can ask for their blood cholesterol level to be ascertained. Appropriate measures can then be taken, if the level is too high, to safeguard future health and this is very likely to include changes being made in the diet.

Hopefully, a consideration of all the factors discussed above can help you to decide whether you need to lose weight in order to safeguard your health, or whether you wish to do so in order to look and feel better about yourself. Additionally or alternatively, you may have decided that it is time to change to a healthier pattern of eating without necessarily expecting a reduction in weight. In fact several diet plans, especially those aiming for a long-term, slow loss of weight, fall more naturally into the latter category. These diet plans are concerned with showing people how to eat healthily so that their weight adjusts to its natural 'set point'. The set point is a person's optimum weight range, which varies around a median level by about ten pounds and is genetically determined. If you are already eating a sensible, healthy diet, are neither fat nor thin and find that your weight does not change very much, then it is likely to lie within the set point range. This factor helps to explain why it can be hard for a dieter to lose the final few pounds to achieve a pre-selected 'target' weight, which may simply have been placed too low for that person's individual set point weight range.

Basal metabolic rate (BMR)
As has been shown, actual weight depends upon a number of different factors, including food intake, lifestyle and amount of physical activity, genes, metabolism, age and existing medical conditions or health problems. The basal metabolic rate (BMR) is the amount of energy (calories) required by the body while at rest to perform the vital functions of heartbeat, respiration, maintenance of body temperature and cellular processes.

Rough calculation of BMR
It can be roughly calculated by multiplying your weight in pounds by a factor of 11, for adults in their twenties. For every decade beyond 20, 2 per cent of the total must be subtracted as this allows for the fact that metabolism slows down with ageing.

Example 1:
For example Suzanne weighs 9 stone 7 lbs and is aged 45:
133 lbs x 11 = 1463
2% of 1463 = 29.26

We now need to subtract 59 [i.e. 2 x 29.26] from 1463, 2% for every decade beyond the twenties.

Suzanne's BMR = 463–59 = <u>1404 kcals per day</u>

Example 2:
Brian weighs 12 stone 4 lbs and is aged 55.
168 lbs x 11 = 1848
2% of 1848 = 36.96

We now need to subtract 111 [i.e. 3 x 36.96] from 1848, 2% for every decade beyond the twenties.

Brian's BMR = <u>1737 kcals per day</u>

The Harris–Benedict Equation for BMR
Other factors can affect the BMR. The last calculation took age into account. Age brings less lean body mass and slows the BMR. Other factors include: the amount of the thyroid hormone thyroxin which is secreted (the more thyroxin the higher the BMR); growth (children and pregnant women have higher BMRs; body composition (the more lean tissue the higher the BMR) environmentatl temperature (heat and cold both raise the BMR).

Another method used to calculate BMR is known as the Harris–Benedict Equation. This takes height and sex into account. Sex is a differential because of the difference in body composition between men and women.

Males: $66 + (13.7 \times W) + (5 \times H) - (6.8 \times A)$
Females: $655 + (9.6 \times W) + (1.7 \times H) - (4.7 \times A)$

W stands for weight in kilograms (weight in pounds divided by 2.2).
H stands for height in centimetres (height in inches x 2.54).
A stands for age in years.

Suzanne weighs 9 stone 7 lbs (133lbs or 60 kg), she is 5 foot 6 inches tall (66 inches or 167.64 cm) and aged 45.

$W = 60$, $H = 167.64$, $A = 45$
$655 + (9.6 \times 60) + (1.7 \times 167) - (4.7 \times 45)$
$655 + 576 + 284 - 211 = \underline{1304 \text{ kcals per day}}$

Suzanne's friend Peter is the same height, weight and age as her but his BMR will be higher because he is a man and men have more lean muscle tissue and less body fat than women.

$66 + (13.7 \times 60) + (5 \times 167) - (6.8 \times 45) = \underline{1584 \text{ kcals per day}}$

Brian weighs 76 kg, is 5 foot 11 inches tall (180.34 cm), and is aged 55.

$66 + (13.7 \times 76) + (5 \times 180) - (6.8 \times 55)$
$66 + 1041.2 + 900 - 374 = \underline{1633.2 \text{ kcals per day}}$

Brian's friend John is the same age and weight but is only 5 foot 3 inches tall. His BMR is 1533 <u>kcals per day</u>.

The above calculations are approximations. Of course, even the most sedentary person requires more calories than the amount demanded by BMR alone. All activity requires energy as fuel, including eating and digesting food – a process which temporarily raises the metabolic rate and burns up some calories to produce heat. Physical activity and regular exercise use up calories but the relationship is a more complex one than many people realize. While exercise plays a crucial part in successful dieting and, most importantly, producing a body that looks and feels good, unless one exercises very hard indeed, it is not a particularly good method of losing weight on its own.

It is known that there is a close relationship between BMR and weight and the heavier the body, the higher the BMR. It is estimated that BMR accounts for about two-thirds of the body's daily need for calories, with the remaining third required for all other activities, just to maintain the person at his or her current weight. Clearly, in order to lose weight, a person needs to eat fewer calories and, as has already been indicated, this may mean nothing more than making adjustments to the diet such as cutting out unnecessary and fattening snacks or second helpings! Many diet plans, especially those aimed at short-term weight loss, are based on a very limited intake of calories. Although this is probably all right for most people for a limited period, it is not a good idea to remain on such a stringent regime for very long. The best diets allow for a gradual return to normal, healthy eating once weight loss has been achieved which will maintain the person at his or her new weight.

Finally, all health experts agree that an average weight loss of 1 to 2 lbs each week should be the aim when dieting. Obviously, the amount of excess weight will determine the overall period of the diet, but it must also be borne in mind that the rate of loss is not uniform. Frequently, a greater amount of weight is lost at the start of a diet than towards the end, so it is necessary to be both patient and persistent. It is always worth remembering that a slow, steady loss of weight is much more likely to result in long-term success, particularly if you remain determined!

Eat Slim

So, as we can see, everyone is individual, and the amount of food each person needs will vary according to individual circumstances: constitution, age, sex, size and activity level. The chart below gives you an approximate idea of the daily calorie intake to aim at for specific weight loss:

Approximate daily calorie intake

Amount to lose	Women	Men (Sedentary/Active)
Up to 6 kg/14 lb	1000	1500/2000
6–12 kg/14–28 lb	1250	1750–2000/2500–2750
Over 12 kg/28 lb	1500	2000–2500/2750–3000

Do not adhere rigidly to these guidelines. Experiment sensibly to see what intake suits you and amend it accordingly. Remember to reduce your intake as the amount of weight to be lost decreases. Remember it is actually more important to be careful about the kinds of calories you consume rather than just the number. Eat healthily.

The following categories have special needs that must be taken into account when calculating calorie intake:

- **Tall people** need more calories than shorter people.
- **Teenagers** need about 20 per cent more and should not have fewer than 1500 calories.
- **Children** need more, relative to their body size. They should

have no fewer than 1500, including a good supply of milk and yoghurt.

- **The elderly** need 10–15 per cent less than the amount listed above. Reductions should be made particularly in foods high in fats and sugar.

Regardless of weight, we are all recommended to consume less fat, sugar and salt, and to eat more fibre. While it *is* possible to lose weight by consuming 1000 calories of chocolate per day, you would soon be suffering from malnutrition – and there is little point in losing weight at the expense of good health. You'd be ravenously hungry too.

If you eat healthily, and by this I mean choosing complex carbohydrates, lean meat, wholemeal grains and pasta, brown rice and pulses, fruit and green vegetables, over highly-processed, quickly-absorbed foods like white bread, fried potatoes, ready-made meals, sugary snacks and cakes, you will feel more full for longer and you may even be able to consume slightly more calories and still lose weight.

Try some of the following tips to help you adjust your eating habits painlessly:

To cut down portions
- Use a smaller plate.
- Eat more slowly, putting your knife and fork down between mouthfuls.
- Take smaller mouthfuls.
- Drink a glass of water or a cup of black tea or coffee about ten minutes before you eat. This will take the edge off your appetite.

To cut down on sugar

- Use artificial sweetener (not cyclamates) in hot drinks and gradually reduce the amount you add.
- Choose low-calorie fizzy drinks rather than the regular variety.
- Add water to fruit juice (it contains a lot of natural sugar).
- Buy sugar-free or low-sugar foods such as baked beans, canned fruit and muesli wherever there is a choice.
- Try having fresh fruit instead of sweets or other sugary snacks.

To cut down on salt

- Add salt at table rather than in cooking – you'll taste it more and thus use less.
- Try using low-sodium salt (half sodium, half potassium) to help you reduce your taste for it.
- Use other flavourings in food: garlic, lemon juice, herbs and spices.
- Avoid foods with high salt content, such as yeast extracts, crisps, peanuts and pickles.

To cut down on fats/cholesterol

- Use low-fat dairy products for spreading, cooking and baking.
- Drink tea and coffee without milk.
- Use low-fat natural yoghurt instead of cream.
- Buy lean cuts of meat.
- Eat more fish.
- Grill rather than fry. If you must fry, use a non-stick pan, which requires less oil.

Counting Calories

- Eat no more than four eggs (boiled or poached) per week.

To increase fibre consumption
- Scrub rather than peel vegetables – the skins are good for you.
- Cook vegetables lightly.
- Eat lots of fresh fruit.
- Buy wholemeal bread, pasta and brown rice.
- Use wholemeal flour for cooking.
- Add beans and grains to soups and stews.

Slimming: Why Bother?

There's no doubt about it – slimming is a demanding, sometimes difficult task, but the benefits are rewarding and sometimes even elating. What will slimming do for you?

It's only natural
Slimness can be seen as the 'natural' state for human beings. Our early ancestors scavenged and hunted for food – an active lifestyle that helped them keep slim. It was only later that 'civilisation' ruined their eating habits – and figures – with over-refined, over-sugary and over-advertised foods.

It's easier . . .
It's easier to romp with the children, to enjoy physical games and exercise, to make love, to run for a bus, to walk the dog . . . and get into a sports car!

It's healthier . . .
Excess weight is associated with high blood pressure, heart disease, stroke, kidney ailments, gallstones, diabetes, varicose veins, gynaecological problems and difficulties with physical co-ordination.

It's worth it!
As one successful slimmer said, 'I didn't know how unfit I was until I lost weight. I just didn't know what I was missing!'

Chubby children
Being fat isn't fun – particularly for children. Playground taunts can be very cruel, and such treatment can sew the seeds

of behaviour in later life – perhaps resulting in an unhappy relationship with food which might lead to anorexia or bulimia (*see* Eating Disorders, page 40).

It's no good making excuses: 'Heaviness runs in the family. We're all on the large size.' It is both unfair and unkind to inflict fatness and your poor eating habits on your children.

Start young with good eating habits and ignore the old adage that a fat baby is a healthy baby – it's not usually true. Serve your children food that is low in fat, sugar and salt, and high in fibre. If they never develop a taste for sugary treats and highly processed foods, they're unlikely to do so in adulthood.

It is a common habit to give food as a reward or for comfort. While this may stop tears or keep children quiet, it is not a good idea on a regular basis. In most instances, a cuddle, a chat or a few minutes of your time to play a game would be just as effective – and calorie-free!

If your children are already overweight, start a healthier approach to food now. Apply all the principles discussed in Eat Slim, Cook Slim and overleaf, and they need never feel deprived or hungry. While it is advisable to keep your children to a healthy eating regime, if your child is overweight you should seek medical advice before putting a diet plan in hand.

Some tips for happy and healthy family meals

- Avoid giving babies food with added sugar. Puddings and rusks frequently contain very high amounts of sugar, so don't serve them. Read labels carefully.

- Give fresh fruit rather than sweets as a snack or treat. There are many exotic varieties to choose from, such as mango, kiwi, tangello and kumquats.

- Make sure your children have a good breakfast and they'll be less likely to snack.
- Always use wholemeal bread – it's more nutritious and more filling.
- Serve favourite foods such as beefburgers, fish fingers and chips only occasionally, choosing the best quality, low-fat varieties available. Grill or oven-bake rather than fry these foods.
- Make your own beefburgers using low-fat mince.
- Buy low-sugar baked beans and ketchup.
- Serve baked potatoes rather than chips.
- Cut down gradually on puddings and offer fresh fruit instead.

Eating Disorders

In any text about slimming, it is important to mention the hazards of taking it too far. Loss of appetite and excessive eating are sometimes symptoms of specific illnesses. For example, it is normal to be 'off your food' if you have 'flu. However, if eating patterns are distorted in otherwise healthy people, they are said to be suffering from eating disorders.

The most serious psychological conditions connected with food and eating in the western world are the eating disorders anorexia nervosa and bulimia nervosa.

Both of these are highly complex conditions which, although centred around food, are in fact manifestations of severe psychological disturbance and distress. Both conditions have become ever more prevalent in recent years, affecting mainly teenagers and young adults and especially girls and young women. Of great concern is the fact that eating disorders are increasingly being reported in children from the age of about 11 years upwards and are not unknown in even younger children. In May 2000, the British Medical Association published a report entitled *Eating Disorders, Body Image and the Media*. The report laid much of the blame for the inexorable rise in these conditions at the door of the fashion and media industries for perpetuating an unhealthy image of thinness, equated with beauty, which is unobtainable for most young women. The fashion industry has hit back by saying that they are now, in fact, using larger models but that in any event, they are only responding to public demand by promoting thinness. Both of these arguments have a very hollow ring to them. Research has shown that the average successful model or actress has only 10 to 15 per cent body fat compared to 22 to

26 per cent for a normal, healthy woman. In order to try to succeed in the world of fashion and media, or to emulate those that do, many young women are going without food and all this at a time when the average size for British women has increased from a 12 to a 14. Also, as discussed previously, it is not the case that ordinary people universally find extreme thinness to be attractive. Surveys consistently reveal that most would prefer to see images of attractive people of average size promoted by the media and that there is a great deal of concern about the rise in incidence of eating disorders.

The power of the media in influencing people's ideas about themselves has been demonstrated by the advent of western television broadcasting to Fiji in 1995. Since western pro- grammes have been shown, there has been an explosion in dieting among Fijian teenagers who were previously not con- cerned about their weight. In Britain, eating disorders con- tinue to exact their toll of suffering upon victims and their families, with both well known and ordinary people being af- fected. In Scotland, there are at least 6000 people suffering from an eating disorder at any particular time and 90 per cent of these are young women. Up to 20 per cent of them die within 20 years from the physical effects of their disorder and even those who survive and are cured can suffer permanent bodily damage.

Anorexia nervosa

The word 'anorexia' means 'loss of appetite', but the disorder is much more complex than that. It is sometimes referred to as 'slimmer's disease', but this term is misleading, for anorexics are more concerned with achieving autonomy than slimness. They often feel helpless and inadequate, even though appear- ing confident.

Anorexics progressively reduce food intake in a pursuit of

thinness that is valued as proof of control rather than as a sign of beauty. It is accompanied by a delusion about true body size and a fear that if normal eating recommences, they will be unable to stop.

It is rare for sufferers to seek help, as they do not usually recognise the syndrome and its dangers. However, they need expert help as soon as possible and should be persuaded to consult a doctor or self-help agency as a matter of urgency (*see also* Further Reading, page 123 and Useful Addresses, page 124).

The characteristic feature of the disorder is that the sufferer has a false and distorted image of herself as being obese, so that when she looks in the mirror she sees a fat person. This generates feelings of disgust and self-loathing and a fear of obesity, amounting to phobia, which renders the victim unable to eat normally. Anorexics are often beset by feelings of shame and secrecy and go to great lengths to conceal their abnormal eating habits and loss of weight from friends and family. If challenged, they deny feeling hunger or that they have a problem and can become quite angry. Self-starvation can be accompanied by excessive exercise, use of laxatives and self-induced vomiting to further promote weight loss. As the weight plummets, menstruation stops, blood pressure falls, there may be vitamin and mineral deficiencies and anaemia, and growth of lanugo – a downy, body hair which the body produces in an attempt to conserve heat and energy. Eventually, body tissues and organs begin to be broken down and there is a serious risk of permanent damage to the heart and sudden death from heart attack. Anorexics commonly suffer from severe depression, some to the point of suicide.

The reasons behind anorexia are complex and while incidence has increased in recent years, evidence suggests that it is a condition which has occasionally arisen throughout history. There is undoubtedly a link with the fashionable and cultural ideal of thinness but it is thought that those who become anorexic are vulnerable in other ways as well. Anorexia commonly develops during adolescence or in the teenage years, at a time when the child is becoming an adult, new feelings and ideas are being experienced and family relationships may be changing. Experts believe that all these factors may be relevant and that anorexia is a reflection of deep psychological insecurity. By denying herself food, the young person may be attempting to somehow reassert control over her life or reverse the process of becoming a sexually functioning adult. Anorexia may also be triggered by profound emotional changes accompanying, for example, separation of parents, bereavement and grief or leaving home.

Whatever the cause, anorexics require specialist help although treatment of the condition can be a prolonged and difficult matter. Specialist residential care and psychotherapy are generally the most successful options but where life is threatened, hospitalization and force feeding may be the only option. Anyone who suspects that a child or friend has anorexia should seek professional help by initially alerting the family doctor, even if the victim herself is uncooperative. Professional support groups exist to help both the victim and her family and the sooner discussion and therapy begin, the sooner progress can be made towards recovery.

Bulimia nervosa

The word 'bulimia' means 'great hunger', but the syndrome is much more complex than that. Massive urges to overeat are built up, which are satisfied by binge-eating. This is followed by efforts to rid the body of the food's potential fattening effects by purging with laxatives or diuretics, by self-induced vomiting or by crash/starvation dieting.

There are links between anorexia and bulimia, and some bulimics (albeit a minority) have previously been anorexics. Consequently, the disorder is also referred to as 'bulimarexia'. The nature of this disorder means that, while eating huge amounts of food, some bulimics remain slim, whilst others undergo wild fluctuations in weight, gaining and losing as much as 45 kg/100 lb between phases of bingeing and purging.

Bulimia is often a secret syndrome accompanied by feelings of shame and disgust. Food is viewed less with pleasure than with fear.

Social pressures to be slim seem to be a major factor in causing bulimia. The fashion for thinness is aided and abetted by an opportunist 'diet industry' promoting the idea that 'thin is beautiful', while advertisers simultaneously extol the delights of fattening foods, and social habits encourage eating almost as a pastime.

The tension and anxiety that these contradictory messages cause may result in people opting for crash or starvation diets in an attempt to get quick results. Such dieting deprives the body of the nutrients it needs and triggers off food cravings. When the tension and/or body's cravings are resolved by binge-eating, bulimia is but a short step away. Initially, slimmers may see the purging that inevitably follows bingeing as a good way of controlling weight gain, but they are often unaware of the disastrous consequences.

The victim is often full of self-disgust, has low self-esteem and tries to conceal her eating habits from others. Bulimia may result in vitamin and mineral deficiencies, gastric problems and ulcers, rotting of teeth and mouth ulcers (caused by stomach acid entering the mouth during frequent vomiting), swelling of joints, disruption of the menstrual cycle, dizziness, headaches, fatigue, abdominal cramps, gum disease, severe constipation, irritability and depression. Most bulimics are able to function normally and maintain a reasonable weight, but in severe and persistent cases, there is a risk of kidney damage, low blood pressure, circulatory problems and dehydration. Bulimia is often accompanied by unhappiness and depression and experts believe that in vulnerable people, it may be triggered by dieting. As with anorexia, it is thought that one of the causes of bulimia is the pressure felt by young people to be thin. The abnormal pattern of eating and purging may arise out of dissatisfaction or hatred of one's body shape and size but may also be a reflection of deeper problems and unhappiness. Anyone who suspects that a family member or friend is suffering from bulimia should try to engage in a sympathetic discussion of the problem and offer support. If the person is cooperative, professional help can be sought through the family doctor which may involve psychotherapy, counselling and possible use of antidepressants. Also, there are support groups which can provide a great deal of help for individual sufferers and their families.Bulimics *must* seek specialist help, either through their GP or a sufferer's support group (*see* Further Reading, page 123 and Useful Addresses, page 124).

Anorexia and bulimia are distressing and damaging disorders but in many cases they can be cured.

The address of the Eating Disorders Association is given on page 124.

Binge eating

A third type of eating disorder affecting obese persons has recently been defined. This is called binge eating disorder and it affects older adults of both sexes in equal numbers. It is characterized by binge eating, but without subsequent misuse of laxatives or induced vomiting and so it may be largely responsible for a person's obesity and lack of success in diet-ing. People suffering from this disorder are often trying to lose weight and are distressed that their lack of control over binge eating which is hindering their efforts to do so. Psycho-therapy and the use of appetite suppressant drugs and possi-bly anti-depressants can help. However, many people remain untreated since the primary problem is seen to be their obes-ity and they may not admit to a disordered pattern of eating. Psychotherapy, along with dietary advice so that the person begins to achieve the desired reduction in weight, seems to offer the best chance of a cure.

Quiz 1:
What Kind of
Thinker are You?

Read the questions and choose (honestly) the answer (A, B, or C) that applies to you.

1 You think you have had a 'good week' of dieting. You get on the scales but you have lost *no* weight. Do you:

A Feel furious and decide it's time to abandon slimming?

B Feel annoyed and promise yourself a treat (food) to console yourself?

C Think critically about everything you *did* eat to see if you could have done better?

2 You have a 'good day' dieting. Then someone offers you a cake, which you eat. Do you:

A Think, 'Oh well, I've blown it. I might as well have another piece?'

B Think, 'That little bit won't hurt?'

C Make up for it by cutting down later – and tomorrow?

3 You see your favourite cream cakes in the baker's window. Do you think:

A 'I want one now' – and have one?

B 'I want one now' – but don't have one?

C This doesn't apply to you – you avoid cake shops.

Counting Calories

4 You read a 'Before and After' story. Do you think:

A 'How marvellous! But I couldn't get as slim as that.'

B 'I think they fake these pictures.'

C 'If she can do it, so can I.'

5 You see a slim, attractive woman whose shape you admire. Do you think:

A 'I bet she can eat anything she likes yet stay slim.'

B 'I wish I was lucky like her.'

C 'I bet she has to work at keeping a shape like that.'

Analysis and Tips

Mostly A answers

These answers indicate negative thinking, characterised by 'I can't', 'I wish' and lack of hope. Negative thought is very destructive to a slimmer's motivation. Worse, it becomes a bad habit, dooming a diet to failure.

You need to:

- **Change** how you think.
- **Monitor** your thoughts. If they are negative, stop and re-phrase them to optimistic ones.
- **Re-read** the C answers in the quiz (the positive ones) and replace your negative thoughts with those.
- **Change** 'I can't' into 'I can' in your thoughts – and you will!

Mostly B answers

These answers indicate 'rationalisation' thoughts. That is, making excuses for behaviour you really know is unhelpful.

You need to:

- **Recognise** that inappropriate eating is always your own responsibility and your own choice.
- **Remind** yourself that excuses can't get you slim – or excuse you.
- **Find** ways other than overeating to reward yourself.

Mostly C answers

These answers indicate positive thinking – the optimism that augurs well for success in slimming.

You need to:

- **Read** both analysis and tips above.
- **Expand** your positive thinking.
- **Re-read** the C (positive) answers in the quiz and use them.

Remember: improve your thinking and you'll improve your slimming.

Quiz 2:
What Kind of
Eater are You?

Answer each question (honestly) with 'yes', 'sometimes' or 'no'. Read the analysis and tips.

Section 1 – Do you:

A Have a snack, a taste or nibble when preparing meals?

B Finish all the food on your plate?

C Have a snack or nibble while watching TV?

D Eat more than you should in restaurants or when eating in other people's houses?

E Find the smell of good food irresistible?

F Eat while standing up or in the car or in rooms of the house other than your dining area?

Section 2 – Do you:

A Eat because you feel unhappy or depressed?

B Eat when you're bored?

C Occasionally get a sudden, uncontrollable urge to eat?

D Eat food that you don't really like if the urge to eat is strong?

E Eat more than usual if you are worried, anxious or under stress?

F Eat when not really hungry if tempting food is offered?

Analysis and tips – Section 1

If you answered 'yes' or 'sometimes' to four or more of these questions, your eating is strongly determined by 'external cues'. This means that the sight and/or smell of food act on you as 'triggers', influencing you to eat too much.

You need to:

- **Reorganise** your life to avoid the sight and smell of food.
- **Keep** all food at home out of sight – tempting treats should be inaccessible, even taped up in containers if necessary.
- **Alter** walking routes to avoid passing tempting shops.
- **Avert** your eyes in the supermarket from 'impulse buy' displays at the checkout.
- **Put** less food on your plate and use a smaller plate.
- **Obey** the rule that you eat *only* when sitting in the dining area at home or work.
- **Never** eat while engaged in another activity.
- **Display** prominently a note: 'Eat for need not greed'.

Analysis and tips – Section 2

If you answered 'yes' or 'sometimes' to four or more of these questions, your eating is strongly determined by your emotions. You may be abusing food as a tranquilliser or anti depressant – eating to solve problems. This fails. It merely gives you another problem – that of excess weight.

You need to:

- **Decide** what the problems are and take action to solve them. Some problems that prompt overeating are stress, marital disharmony, sexual problems, depression, anxiety, boredom and anger (maybe repressed). Women may also have physical problems connected with periods, contraception or the menopause. If you suspect that these, or any other problems, are at the root of your overeating, do not despair – self-help is often possible. *See* Further Reading, page 123 and Useful Addresses, page 124, for starting points.

- **Try** classes in relaxation, yoga and/or exercise.
- **Keep** repeating to yourself: 'Eating doesn't solve problems, it only makes me fat.'
- **Seek** medical help if your weight is making you anxious.
- **Find** other ways of rewarding yourself.

Other scores

If you have 'yes' answers in both sections, you need to tackle both angles as suggested above. All 'no' answers? Were you being honest?

Health and Nutrition

In recent years it has been realised that good health, as well as a slim figure, is not so much a matter of luck as a matter of what we choose to eat.

Food is the 'fuel' that keeps the body in good working order and supplies the energy for all activities. It is composed of many different nutrients, each of which performs a different function in the body. As very few foods contain *all* the nutrients necessary for good health, it is important to eat a variety of foods to ensure a balanced diet. There are five categories of food essential to health and vitality:

1 Protein
This is used for building, maintenance and repair of body tissues. In children and teenagers it is also used for growth. Protein should be eaten every day and constitute 10–15 per cent of your daily calorie intake (50 g/2 oz for women and 90 g/ 3.5 oz for men, depending on how active the lifestyle).

There is little point in eating more protein than you require, as it is simply expelled in the urine or stored as fat. Good, low-fat sources of protein include poultry, white fish, eggs, soya products, cottage cheese and yoghurt. Other less rich sources include cereals, bread, rice, potatoes and pulses.

2 Carbohydrates
These are divided into three types: sugars, starches and fibre.

Sugar
Sugar occurs naturally in certain foods, for example, fructose in fruit and lactose in milk. Refined sugar (sucrose), used in

tea, coffee, biscuits and sweets, is an 'empty' food: it has no nutrients at all so it is completely superfluous to dietary needs. Consuming sweet things raises the blood sugar level very quickly but it drops again equally rapidly, so you still feel hungry and may even develop a craving for more sweet things. For these reasons you should avoid sugar or keep it to a minimum.

Starch

Starch is a tasteless white substance found in many foods such as bread, potatoes, pasta, rice, cereals and beans. It tends to be bulky, so is useful for making the stomach feel full.

Fibre

Sometimes called 'roughage', fibre is an indigestible carbohydrate that cannot be absorbed by the body. It simply passes through the digestive tract, helping its efficiency and reducing the risk of constipation and disease. Fibre is good news for slimmers as, when consumed with liquid, it helps to fill you up so you eat less. (Note that high-fibre diets *must* be accompanied by lots of liquid – at least 1.7–2.2 litres/3–4 pints a day.) The recommended daily fibre intake for adults is about 30 g/1.25 oz. Good sources of fibre include bran cereals, sugar-free muesli, wholemeal products, jacket potatoes, lightly cooked vegetables, pulses and fruit (with skin when possible).

In their natural, unrefined state carbohydrates are an important source of energy and nutrition. They should account for 55–60 per cent of your daily calorie intake. Like any food, if you eat more than your body requires the excess is stored as fat.

3 Fats and oils

These may be divided into three types: saturates, mono-unsaturates and polyunsaturates. All fats contain a mixture of the three so they are labelled according to which type predominates.

Saturates

Saturates, found in dairy products, meat (especially red), hard fats and coconut oil, are not an essential part of the diet. In fact, they are believed to cause an accumulation of cholesterol in the blood which 'furs' the arteries and can lead to heart attacks. It is generally agreed that we should all avoid saturated fats and minimise consumption of high-cholesterol foods such as egg yolks and liver.

Monounsaturates

Monounsaturates are present in olive oil, nuts and seeds, and should be consumed in preference to saturates.

Polyunsaturates

Polyunsaturates are the only fats the body actually needs because they contain two essential fatty acids that cannot be synthesised by the body. However, the requirement is a mere 40 g/1.5 oz per day. Make sure the fats and oils you buy are labelled 'high in polyunsaturates'.

Given these facts, most people can afford to cut fat intake considerably. Weight for weight, fats have a higher calorific value than any other food so they should be kept to a minimum in any slimming diet. Remember that some foods have a 'hidden' fat content: cakes, biscuits, pastries, ice-cream, chocolate and meat (even when visible fat has been removed). Try to avoid all these things and use low-fat substitutes whenever possible.

4 Vitamins

These enable the body to process foods so they can do their jobs properly. Fat-soluble vitamins (A, D, E and K) are stored in the liver and fatty tissues, but water-soluble vitamins (B group, C and folic acid) cannot be stored for long so adequate amounts must be eaten every day.

Vitamin A

Found in carrots, liver, milk, butter, margarine, egg yolk, cheese, tomatoes, dark green vegetables, yellow and orange fruits, halibut and cod liver oils.

The B vitamins

- *1 (thiamin)* – found in milk, lean bacon, pork, cod's roe, liver, kidney, pulses, peanuts, oatmeal, flour and bread, brewer's yeast, wheatgerm, enriched breakfast cereals.
- *B_2 (riboflavin)* – found in milk, yoghurt, cheese, liver, kidney, egg, bran, brewer's yeast, curd cheese.
- *B_3 (niacin)* – found in peanuts, peanut butter, wholemeal bread, brewer's yeast, meat, liver, coffee, beer, pulses, yeast extract, potatoes, enriched cereals.
- *B_6 (pyridoxine)* – found in potatoes, leafy vegetables, whole grains and cereals, nuts, fresh and dried fruits.
- *B_{12}* – found in liver, heart, sardines, cheese, eggs, milk.

Folic acid

Found in liver, fish, avocados, green vegetables, wholemeal bread, eggs, bananas, oranges, bran, beetroot, peanuts.

Vitamin C

Found in all fresh fruits and vegetables but can be drastically reduced by prolonged cooking or storage. Good sources include blackcurrants, greens, raw cabbage, gooseberries, citrus fruits, guava, parsley, green and red peppers, sprouts, watercress.

Vitamin D
Found in herrings, kippers, salmon, sardines, mackerel and pilchards, egg yolks, margarine, butter and liver. It is also produced by the action of sunlight on the skin.

Vitamin E
Found in dark green vegetables, wheatgerm, vegetable oils, whole grains, nuts, eggs.

Vitamin K
Found in leafy vegetables, yoghurt, egg yolks.

5 Minerals
These do not mean a lot to most people, but they are vital to well-being. Among the essentials are:

Calcium
Found in dairy products, sardines, soya beans, molasses, broccoli, peanuts and white bread. Women and girls should have up to 500 mg daily to lessen the risk of osteoporosis in later life.

Iodine
Found in seafood, milk, eggs, meat, vegetables.

Iron
Found in liver, kidney, beef, wholemeal bread, potatoes, watercress, dried apricots and soy sauce. Menstruating women and girls need a good supply of iron to lessen the chances of becoming anaemic.

Magnesium
Found in vegetables and grains.

Phosphorus
Found in nuts, eggs, soya and whole grains.

Potassium
Found in milk, vegetables and fruit.

Sodium
Found in most vegetables, often added as salt.

Zinc
Found in milk, hard cheeses, wholemeal bread, meat, offal and shellfish, especially oysters.

Water
Water is also essential to every bodily process. You should aim to drink around 1.75 litres/3 pints a day, whether bottled, straight from the tap or in the form of tea, coffee or low-calorie drinks. Excess liquid is not stored as fat; it is simply expelled in the urine.

Planning your Eating

Most people, including slimmers, eat three meals a day: breakfast, a light meal and a main meal. It does not matter whether you choose to eat your main meal at lunch or dinner. The important thing is to organise your eating to suit your lifestyle.

If you like to eat little but often, you can divide your daily food allowance into five smaller snack meals. Studies have suggested that more weight can be lost using this system than eating the same amount of food divided into three meals. Try it and see if it works for you.

However you choose to organise your eating, always keep the following points in mind:

- Eat at regular intervals. This benefits your body and avoids lengthy gaps between meals which may trigger snacking or a binge later.

- Weigh ingredients and portions. Estimating inevitably leads to overestimating and thus overeating.

- Use leftovers as the basis of another meal or throw them away. Do not finish them up yourself, even if you hate the thought of wasting good food.

- Do not eat later than nine o'clock. It's uncomfortable to go to bed with a full stomach and, more importantly, your body cannot burn off the calories so efficiently.

Breakfast: A Good Way to Start the Day

Many slimmers eat no breakfast. It seems an easy meal to miss, and calories can be saved, but it is unwise to do so. The body has 'fasted' all night and its blood sugar levels are low.

A balanced breakfast starts up the bodily system and helps us feel more awake and energetic, better able to cope with the morning. The slimmer who eats breakfast is less likely to turn to mid-morning snacks as a crutch or comfort. Those who miss breakfast will often find themselves craving something sweet, or even bingeing, later on. This craving is not because of poor willpower but a physiological need. It is the body's response to being deprived of the nutrients it needs. The awakening body is functioning at its lowest metabolic rate (i.e. the rate at which it burns up food into energy). The lower that rate remains, the slower food is burned up and, therefore, the slower any weight loss. The very act of eating is believed to raise the metabolic rate (the 'thermogenic effect') so breakfast can be good for those wanting to maximise weight loss.

What's for Breakfast?

As with any other meal, your choice of food is crucial. Consider the information and tips given in the Health and Nutrition section and Eat Slim: aim to minimise fats and avoid refined sugar.

The six breakfast ideas below could easily be incorporated into a woman's diet of 1000 calories per day. Men in sedentary jobs may increase the amounts by half, while highly active men or manual workers may double them.

One
25 g/1 oz high-fibre cereal
125 ml/ ¼ pint skimmed milk or low-fat yoghurt
  or fruit (fresh or tinned, no added sugar)

Two
1 slice bacon
1 grilled tomato

1 egg
25 g/1 oz bread
Three
75 g/3 oz cottage cheese
2 slices crispbread or 50 g/2 oz bread or toast

Four

50 g/2 oz toast
2 tomatoes and/or mushrooms

Five

1 low-fat yoghurt
$1/2$ chopped apple
$1/2$ chopped banana
(substitute other fresh fruit if preferred)

Six

50 g/2 oz wholemeal toast
15 g/$1/2$ oz low-fat spread
Tea or coffee, served black with lemon or skimmed milk,
would complete a nutritious but low-calorie start to the day.

Light Meals and Snacks

Snacks

There should really be no need to snack if you're eating sensible meals, but in the first few days of a diet you may experience hunger pangs while your stomach is adjusting to a lower food intake.

A glass of water or cup of tea will help to fill you up, but if you really must nibble, have a supply of celery and carrot sticks in the fridge and keep the fruit bowl topped up.

Counting Calories

Light meals

What is a light meal? For some it could be an orange, for others it could be fish and chips. Keeping in mind your calorie allowance, a light meal should be satisfying enough to keep you from snacking between meals and fulfil all the criteria outlined in the Health and Nutrition section.

Below are some ideas for light meals that are nutritious and low in calories:

Sandwiches

These are as good for you as what goes into them. Ideally, make them at home with wholemeal bread and low-fat spread or low-calorie mayonnaise. If you use a moist filling, you can omit the spread or mayonnaise completely and save a few calories.

To save time (and to avoid impulse overeating if you are at home all day), make a batch of sandwiches, divide them into small packs and put them in the refrigerator, ready to eat as required.

Purchased sandwiches may exceed 450 calories per slice, so avoid them if possible. If you do buy some, have them freshly made up with no butter, margarine or mayonnaise.

Low-calorie sandwich fillings

- 50 g/2 oz tuna (tinned in brine, not oil) mixed with a little chopped onion
- 25 g/1 oz mackerel (tinned in brine, not oil) mixed with a little low-calorie salad cream or mayonnaise
- 25 g/1 oz grated low-fat cheese with tomato and onion or sweet pickle or piccalilli
- 50 g/2 oz prawns mixed with low-calorie seafood dressing and lettuce

- 50 g/2 oz skinned, cooked chicken mixed with chopped onion and low-calorie salad cream or mayonnaise. If you like,
  add a little tandoori spice to the dressing.

Accompany your sandwiches with homemade coleslaw in
low-calorie dressing. Finish your meal with one piece of fresh
fruit of your choice.

Jacket potatoes

The humble potato is a good source of nutrition and fibre
and can make a satisfying meal. Choose one weighing about
150 g/5 oz and try it with one of the fillings suggested:

Low-calorie potato fillings

- 75 g/3 oz cottage cheese
- 25 g/1 oz grated low-fat hard cheese with tomato and
  chopped onion
- 50 g/2 oz low-sugar baked beans
- 50 g/2 oz prawns with low-calorie mayonnaise

Omelettes

Eggs are endlessly versatile and lend themselves to quick,
warming meals. For a low-calorie omelette, mix together two
eggs with a little skimmed milk and fry in a non-stick pan
without fat. Remember to limit your weekly egg consumption to no more than four. For added flavour try the omelette
with one of the following:

- 25 g/1 oz chopped lean ham
- 2 chopped tomatoes
- 50 g/2 oz sliced mushrooms
- 1 tablespoon fresh chopped herbs, such as chives

Counting Calories

Soup
Homemade soups tend to be rather calorific (though they needn't be) and may not always be to hand. For a light meal, use a packet of low-calorie soup in the flavour of your choice. To make it more interesting, add some chopped vegetables (not potatoes) either raw or cooked.

Main Meals
Your main meal of the day should be based on protein food, preferably fish or poultry. Red meats contain a lot of hidden fat so choose lean pork rather than beef or lamb: it's less fattening.

To save time, you could prepare double quantities of such dishes as casseroles, chilli con carne and curry, freezing half for future use. Alternatively, keep a stock of purchased low-calorie meals. Although these can be expensive, they are convenient and can be served with lightly cooked fresh vegetables for a balanced meal.

Slimmers must abandon the traditional three-course main meal except for special occasions or a weekend treat. Restrict the meal to one main course and have fresh fruit or yoghurt instead of a pudding. On the occasions when a first course is needed, have low-calorie soup or melon.

Remember, food does not have to be hot to constitute a 'proper' meal. Cold lean meat and salad, for example, can be both satisfying and nutritious. Add a hot baked potato if you wish.

Read and put into practice the tips given in Eat Slim, page 33, and Cook Slim, page 71, then try some of the main meal ideas.

Satisfying and slimming
• Lean roast pork, lamb or beef with boiled potatoes and

vegetables (75 g/3 oz meat per woman and 100–125 g/4–5 oz per man)

- Skinless roast chicken or turkey with chosen vegetables (10 g/4 oz meat per woman and 125–150 g/5–6 oz per man)
- Grilled pork or lamb chop with baked potato and chosen vegetables (the chop should weigh 125 g/5 oz per woman and 150–175 g/6–7 oz per man)
- Lamb or pork chop casserole with onions and mushrooms and sliced potato on top (quantities as above)
- Chicken or lamb's liver casserole with onions, mushrooms and tomatoes (quantities as roast pork)
- Cod in white, parsley or onion sauce made with skimmed milk (150 g/6 oz per woman, 175–200g/7–8 oz per man)
- Hot or cold peppered mackerel with horseradish sauce, baked potato, peas, sweetcorn and/or coleslaw
- Wholemeal pasta dishes, such as lasagne, with a green salad
- Low-calorie prepared meals of 400 calories or fewer each. Serve with lightly cooked vegetables
- Stir-fry packs are quick and easy. Cook with water or two teaspoons of polyunsaturated oil. You can 'stretch' the pack for two people by adding chopped fresh vegetables, part-cooked brown rice and, if necessary, some cooked chopped meat
- French bread pizza, made by several frozen food manufacturers, can be served with low-calorie coleslaw or fresh vegetables

Remember: boredom is an enemy of the slimmer. Make your meals interesting and you'll be more successful in sticking to your diet.

'Safer' Shopping

It can be very daunting to the willpower to be confronted with so many temptations while shopping, particularly in supermarkets. If you really want to avoid buying food with a high calorific value, there are a few simple rules you can follow:

- **Avoid** shopping when you feel hungry – you will be tempted to buy fattening snacks.
- **Take** a shopping list with you – and stick to it.
- **Write out** the shopping list while you are *not* hungry.
- **Take** a low-calorie snack with you in case you are delayed. (A piece of crispbread, celery or carrot would suffice.)
- **Carry** powdered skimmed milk in an empty tablet bottle to add to tea or coffee when out.
- **Take** a flask of ready-made tea or coffee on outings to quieten hunger pangs and stave off impulse eating.
- **Avoid** passing confectionery shelves or shops if possible.
- **Discourage** your children from eating sweets. This will protect *their* teeth from decay and *you* from temptation.
- **Read** food labels for calorie content and avoid products with added sugar. Even savoury products can contain sugar, so be selective.
- **Don't** buy 'economy' packs of chocolate or sugary treats; you know the economy turns to temptation once you get the pack home.
- **Inform** the store manager if the diet foods you want are not in stock.

Understanding food labels

By law, all food labels must show a complete list of the product's ingredients in descending order of weight. If, for example, sugar appears high in the list of ingredients, you know that the product contains quite a lot of it.

Unfortunately, additional laws making it compulsory to give other nutritional information are, as yet, only under consideration.

Don't be daunted by food labels – they're easy to understand once you have a little practice.

Nutrition

In addition to these ingredients, most labels list any additives the product contains. These frequently appear as E numbers. If you wish to find out more about additives, *see* Further Reading, page 123.

Finally, beware products labelled 'suitable for diabetics' and vague claims such as 'all natural'. Although diabetic foods contain no sugar, they have a high-calorie substitute so they are not advantageous to slimmers. Similarly, claims about the 'natural' content of food does not preclude it having large amounts of sugar or saturated fat, both of which are naturally occurring substances.

Slimmer's shopping list

The slimmer's shopping list and store cupboard must be adapted to cater for new and healthier eating habits. Most of the items listed below are staples so they are occasional rather than weekly buys. Substitute them for your usual items in each category. Remember: convenience foods are not necessarily junk foods. If in doubt, read the labels for sugar and fat content.

Counting Calories

Dairy produce
- skimmed milk
- low-fat spread to replace butter and margarine
  (Note that margarines labelled 'high in polyunsaturates' are not low-calorie unless stated)
- low-fat, sugar-free yoghurt
- Smetana/low-fat sour cream to replace ordinary cream
- low-fat hard cheeses
- low-fat soft cheeses
- low-fat cheese spreads
- low-fat processed cheese slices

Breakfast cereals
- All-Bran
- Grape Nuts
- muesli mixture with no added sugar
- Nutrigrain

Main meals
- fish without batter or sauce
- seafood such as prawns and mussels
- vegetables (freezing retains their vitamins and minerals)
- calorie-counted frozen meals
- skinless chicken pieces
- pre-packed mackerel, peppered or with mustard
- avoid processed and high-fat foods, such as beefburgers, sausages and meat pies, where the quality of the meat is uncertain and the proportion of fat to meat is usually high.

Dry goods

- brown rice
- dried fruit
- wholemeal pasta
- pulses (beans, lentils, peas)
- wholemeal flour

Tinned goods

- tuna and mackerel in brine, not oil
- salmon, especially Keta
- tomatoes
- low-sugar baked beans
- sugar-free corn kernels
- pulses (e.g. chickpeas and kidney beans) – they need no soaking
- low-calorie soups
- fruit in natural juice or water, not syrup

Condiments

- low-calorie salad cream and mayonnaise
- oil-free salad dressing
- low-calorie vinaigrette
- low-calorie seafood dressing

Spreads

- low-fat pâté (available in some supermarkets)
- low-sugar jams
- yeast extracts (use sparingly as they are high in salt)

Herbs, spices and flavourings

Add extra interest to your cooking with some of the huge range of herbs, spices and flavourings currently available. You may well have a selection of the following items in stock already, so try some of the unusual ones just for a change:

- **Herbs and spices:** basil, bay leaves, cardamom, cayenne pepper, chillies, chives, cinnamon, cloves, coriander, cumin, curry powder (preferably homemade), garlic/garlic granules, ginger, juniper, marjoram, nutmeg, oregano, paprika, parsley, rosemary, saffron, sage, tarragon, thyme, turmeric.

- **Flavourings:** black peppercorns, linseeds, mustards, sesame seeds, soy sauce, Tabasco sauce, vinegars (wine, cider, fruit, herb, balsamic), Worcestershire sauce.

- Try to minimise your use of salt and sugar. If necessary use a low-sodium salt substitute and a low-calorie sweetener.

Drinks

- decaffeinated coffee (available in fresh and instant forms)
- low-calorie mixers, such as lemonade and ginger ale
- mineral waters (sparkling and still)
- fruit and herb teas
- Avoid fruit juices as they are high in natural sugars. Also avoid fruit 'drinks', which always contain added sugar.

Cook Slim

If you follow the advice in Eat Slim and 'Safer' Shopping, you're probably buying good food that is reasonably low in calories. However, it is essential to prepare it in a low-calorie way so that your sensible purchases don't turn into a dieting disaster.

Being the only slimmer in the household does not mean that you have to eat in isolation. In fact, the family need never know that you're trying to lose weight. They will all benefit from the low-fat, low-sugar, high-fibre approach to cooking, and your efforts can reap health dividends for everyone, decreasing excess weight where necessary and giving protection against a variety of diet-related illnesses, especially heart disease.

Food preparation
- **Cut off** all visible fat from meat.
- **Remove** all skin from poultry *before* cooking.
- **Weigh,** do not guess, your portions.
- **Scrub** rather than peel vegetables.
- **Avoid** nibbling.

Useful equipment
Old habits need not die hard. Use some of the items below in order to save nutritional content and minimise the use of fat in cooking:
- **Steamer** – for fish and vegetables. This is clean and easy to use although it is slower than boiling or baking. However, as the food is not sitting in water, valuable vitamins and minerals cannot leak out.

Counting Calories

- **Wok** – an ancient but highly efficient cooking implement that requires only a tiny amount of oil or water for cooking. Its shape helps to spread the heat quickly and evenly so food can cook in minutes and thus retain its nutritional content.
- **Food processor** – invaluable for chopping up vegetables, particularly for coleslaw.
- **Microwave cooker** – great for baked potatoes, the hungry slimmer's healthy fast food.

Cooking methods

- Dry-fry in a non-stick pan whenever possible. If a recipe specifies pre-frying ingredients, simply miss out this step – you won't notice the difference in the finished dish. If you insist on frying, use two teaspoons of polyunsaturated oil, such as sunflower or rapeseed.
- Minced beef usually contains quite a lot of fat, so it may be dry-fried and the fat drained off before continuing with the recipe.
- Grill, poach, steam, bake, pressure-cook or microwave in preference to frying or roasting whenever possible.
- Avoid deep-frying. If you must cook chips, cut them straight and chunky, not thin or crinkly, so that they absorb less fat. All deep-fried foods should be a very occasional treat.
- Thicken casseroles by draining off the liquid and fast-boiling it to reduce. (Thickeners, such as cornflour or gravy granules, add lots of extra calories.)
- Avoid tasting dishes too often. Three or four spoonfuls of a sauce or gravy can contain a surprising number of calories. If you must taste, use a teaspoon.

Healthy subsitutions

- Skimmed milk instead of whole milk in drinks, sauces, custard, milk puddings, mashed potatoes and scrambled eggs.
- Low-fat natural yoghurt for cream in casseroles and cake fillings. (Add it at the last minute to hot dishes to prevent it curdling.)
- Sorbet or yoghurt ice-cream instead of regular ice-cream or custard.
- Wholemeal pasta and brown rice for white varieties – they're more filling
- Wholemeal flour for white, or use half and half.
- Low-fat spread for butter and margarine.
- Jacket potatoes for chips and boiled potatoes.
- Low-fat roast potatoes for traditional ones (Cut larger, but fewer, chunks, brush lightly with oil and cook in a lightly oiled roasting tin.)

Be open-minded about trying new dishes. Train yourself to unaccustomed flavours with small 'tasters' and experiment with different herbs and spices. There is no need to bore yourself with dull or repetitive food.

Try to adapt your favourite recipe with the Cook Slim guidelines in mind. If you're stuck for inspiration, borrow or buy some new cookbooks that specialise in low-fat, low-sugar cuisine (*see* Further Reading, page 123). You'll soon discover that meals can be delicious as well as low-calorie and nutritious.

Entertaining

All the Cook Slim tips should be applied when planning to entertain, whether for a small dinner party or a banquet for hundreds. With care and imagination, you can produce dishes that taste so good that your guests will never believe they're low-calorie and healthy.

The following tips may help the occasion to go smoothly:

- **Offer** guests a selection of alcoholic and non-alcoholic drinks. Don't forget to have low-calorie mixers for yourself and other slimmers.

- **Canapés** can be highly calorific. If you want to serve 'nibbles', prepare some crudités and low-calorie dips.

- **Minimise** meal preparation time by choosing a cold starter and a cold dessert. For starters you could have melon balls and black grapes in port, pink grapefruit with prawns, or prawn cocktail with low-calorie seafood dressing. For dessert you could have fresh fruit salad, individual meringues topped with raspberries or other soft fruit, sorbet or low-calorie trifle.

- **Choose** dishes that contrast in colour, texture and flavour. This sounds obvious but it's a common mistake to combine dishes that are too similar to each other. For example, avoid serving a lemon mousse for dessert if you intend having a fish mousse starter.

- **Serve** mineral water as well as wine with the meal so that drivers, slimmers and teetotallers are catered for.

Preparing low-calorie dinner parties

Starters

Choose	Avoid
melon	avocado
crudités	anything fried or coated in oil, oil-based dressings or mayonnaise
sorbet	creamy soups
prawns	

Main courses

Choose	*Avoid*
poultry	anything fried
white fish	rich, creamy sauces
lean meat	batter or suet puddings
lobster	pastry dishes – pies and quiches
steamed vegetables	buttered vegetables
mixed salads dressed in yoghurt with lemon juice and herbs	

Desserts

Choose	Avoid
sorbet	fritters
fresh fruit	cream
unsweetened fruit salad	gateaux
	choux pastry
fruit fools made with yoghurt, and no added sugar	fruit fools made with custard and cream
	pies
	puddings
	meringues

Low-calorie Recipes

Here are some basic recipes that demonstrate the principles of making low-calorie versions of some favourite foods.

Coleslaw
white cabbage
onion
low-calorie mayonnaise, oil-free
    dressing or low-calorie seafood
    dressing
few drops lemon juice

Chop the cabbage and onion into thin shreds, either by hand or in a food processor. Mix in your chosen dressing and serve. Try adding chopped carrot, celery, cucumber or cauliflower to the basic mixture – you'll soon find your favourite combination.

Chicken risotto
125 g/4 oz brown rice
125 g/4 oz frozen sweetcorn ker-
    nels
2 tsp polyunsaturated oil or 1 tbsp
    water
1 small onion, chopped
1 small clove garlic or 1 tsp garlic
    granules (optional)
1 tsp mild curry powder (optional)
397 g/14 oz can tomatoes
few cauliflower or broccoli florets
175 g/6 oz cooked chicken

Boil the rice. When nearly done, boil the sweetcorn. Heat the oil or water in a non-stick pan and fry the onion until soft, not brown. Add the garlic and curry powder and cook over a gentle heat for a few minutes. Add the tomatoes, cauliflower, drained sweetcorn and chicken. Heat thoroughly for about 7 minutes, then stir in the rice. Serve with wholemeal bread.

Chilli casserole

500g/1 lb lean stewing beef, cut
    into 2 cm/1 inch cubes
1 medium onion, sliced
397 g/14 oz can red kidney beans,
    drained and rinsed
200 g/7 oz can low-sugar baked beans
1 tsp chilli powder
285 ml/1 pint beef stock

Heat the oven to 170°C (325°F or gas mark 3). Place all the ingredients in a casserole. Cover and cook slowly for 2–2$\frac{1}{2}$ hours. Remove cover, strain off liquid and boil to reduce to desired consistency. Return to casserole and serve.

Seafood dip

150 g/5 oz low-fat natural yoghurt
3 level tbsp low-calorie seafood
    dressing
pinch pepper
1$\frac{1}{2}$ level tsp creamed horseradish
    (optional)

Combine all the ingredients by hand or in a food processor.

Cheese, onion and garlic dip

150 g/5 oz low-fat natural yoghurt
3 level tbsp low-calorie blue
 cheese dressing
75 g/3 oz chopped onion
1 clove garlic, crushed, or 50 g/2 oz
 chopped cucumber (optional)

Combine all the ingredients by hand or in a food processor.

Lean-line lasagne

350 g/12 oz lean or low-fat minced
 beef
1 tsp polyunsaturated oil or $1/2$ tsp
 water (optional)
1 medium onion, chopped
1 small green pepper, seeded and
 chopped
4 sticks celery, chopped
125 g/4 oz mushrooms, sliced
397 g/14 oz can tomatoes
2 cloves garlic, crushed, or 1 tsp
 garlic granules
$1/2$ tsp mixed herbs
$1/2$ tsp oregano
pinch cayenne pepper
1 stock cube, crumbled
125 g/4 oz wholewheat lasagne (no
 pre-cooking variety)
25 g/1 oz cornflour
$1/2$ tsp mustard
pinch pepper
568 ml/1 pint skimmed milk

40 g/1¹/₂ oz Edam or low-fat hard
cheese, grated

Brown the meat in a non-stick pan with or without the oil or
water. Drain off any fat from the meat. Add the onion, green
pepper, celery, mushrooms, tomatoes, garlic, herbs, cayenne
and stock cube to the pan. Bring to the boil, then cover and
simmer for 45 minutes, removing the lid for the last 10 minutes. Place half the meat mixture in an ovenproof dish and
cover with half the lasagne. Repeat. Heat the oven to 200°C
(400°F or gas mark 6). Mix the cornflour, mustard and pepper with a little of the milk to form a smooth paste. Pour the
remaining milk into a saucepan, stir in the cornflour paste
and bring to the boil, stirring continuously. Cook gently for 1
minute. Stir in half the cheese. When melted, pour the sauce
over the lasagne. Sprinkle the remaining cheese on top and
bake for about 50 minutes.

*Variation: Replace the meat with a mixture of vegetables, such
as cauliflower, broccoli, carrots, sweetcorn, peas, leeks or kidney
beans.*

Pasta spirals with lemon sauce and dill
250 g/8 oz pasta spirals
¹/₄ litre/8 fl oz milk
¹/₈ tsp salt
4 tbsp aquavit or 4 tbsp vodka and
1 tsp caraway seeds
3 tbsp fresh lemon juice
5 cm/2 inch strip of lemon rind
2 tbsp finely cut fresh dill or 2 tsp
dried dill

Put the milk, salt, aquavit or vodka and caraway seeds, lemon
juice and lemon rind in a large non-stick or heavy frying pan.

Bring the liquid to the boil, reduce the heat and simmer gently for 3 minutes. Add the spirals and enough water to almost cover them. Cover the pan and cook over low heat, removing the lid and stirring occasionally, until the spirals are *al dente* and about 4 tablespoons of sauce remains – approximately 15 minutes. (If necessary, add more water to keep the spirals from sticking.) Remove the lemon rind and discard it. Stir in the chopped dill and serve the dish immediately

Spaghetti with smoked salmon and watercress

250 g/8 oz spaghetti
$1^1/_2$ tsp virgin olive oil
1 garlic clove, finely chopped
60 g/2 oz smoked salmon, julienned
1 bunch watercress, washed and stemmed
freshly ground black pepper

Cook the spaghetti in 3 litres (5 pints) of boiling water with $1^1/_2$ teaspoons of salt. Start testing the pasta after 8 minutes and cook it until it is *al dente*. Just before the spaghetti finishes cooking, heat the oil in a large frying pan over medium heat. Cook the garlic in the oil for 30 seconds, stirring constantly. Add the salmon, watercress and pepper, and cook for 30 seconds more before removing the pan from the heat. Drain the spaghetti and add it to the pan. Toss the spaghetti to distribute the sauce and serve at once.

Courgette tian

750 g/$1^1/_2$ lb courgettes, trimmed and finely sliced
3 tsp virgin olive oil

60 g/2 oz brown rice
1 garlic clove
$1/4$ tsp salt
3 shallots, finely chopped
2 small eggs, beaten
2 tbsp freshly grated Parmesan
  cheese
1 tbsp shredded fresh rocket
  leaves
1 tbsp shredded fresh basil leaves
1 tbsp finely chopped flat-leaf
  parsley
$1/8$ tsp white pepper

Place the courgettes in a heavy-bottomed saucepan with 2 teaspoons of the oil and cook them gently over low heat, covered, until they are just tender – about 10 minutes. Stir from time to time to prevent the courgettes from sticking.

Rinse the brown rice under cold running water and place it in a small, heavy-bottomed saucepan with 30 cl ($1/2$ pint) of water. Bring the water to the boil, reduce the heat, cover the pan and simmer for 15 minutes. Drain the rice well and set it aside, covered.

Preheat the oven to 180°C (350°F or gas mark 4). Crush the garlic with the salt. Heat the remaining teaspoon of oil in a small, heavy-bottomed saucepan, add the shallots and garlic, and soften them over very low heat, covered, for about 5 minutes.

Lightly grease a wide, shallow gratin dish. In a large mixing bowl, stir together the courgettes, rice, shallots and garlic. Add the eggs and half the Parmesan. Stir well, then mix in the rocket, basil, parsley and pepper. Transfer the mixture to the prepared dish, levelling the courgette slices so that they lie flat, and sprinkle on the remaining Parmesan.

Bake the tian in the oven, uncovered, for 20 minutes, then increase the oven temperature to 220°C (425°F or gas mark 7) and bake it for a further 10 to 15 minutes until a crust has formed.

Serve hot or warm.

Red-cooked beef

1 kg/2 lb topside of beef, trimmed of fat and cut into 2 cm ($^3/_4$ inch) pieces

4 Chinese dried mushrooms, soaked in hot water for 10 to 15 minutes

3 tbsp low-sodium soy sauce or shoyu

2 tbsp dry sherry

2 tbsp soft brown sugar

1 tbsp tomato paste

2.5 cm/1 inch fresh ginger root, peeled and crushed

2 garlic cloves, crushed

$^1/_2$ tsp five-spice powder

$^1/_4$ litre/8 fl oz unsalted brown stock

1 tbsp safflower oil

300 g/10 oz carrots, thinly sliced diagonally

Drain the mushrooms and gently squeeze out excess moisture. Trim and slice them. Place them in a bowl with the soy sauce or shoyu, sherry, brown sugar, tomato paste, ginger, garlic, five-spice powder and stock. Stir well and set aside.

Heat the oil in a heavy, fireproof casserole over high heat. Add one third of the beef pieces and brown them on all sides, turning them constantly – about 5 minutes. With a slotted spoon, drain the meat, then transfer it to a plate lined with paper towels. Repeat with the remaining two batches of beef, draining each batch on fresh towels. Return all the beef to the casserole, add the mushrooms and liquid mixture and bring slowly to the boil Reduce the heat, cover and simmer very gently for $1^1/_2$ hours, turning the meat over frequently during this time and basting with the cooking liquid.

Add the carrots and continue cooking for a further 30 minutes or until the beef is tender; the carrots should be cooked but still firm. Serve hot.

Braised chicken with plums and lemons

4 chicken breasts, skinned and
    boned (about 500 g/1 lb)
$^1/_2$ litre/16 fl oz unsalted chicken
    stock
4 red plums, blanched in the stock
    for 1 minute, peeled (skins re-
    served), halved and stoned
2 tsp sugar
30 g/1 oz unsalted butter
$^1/_8$ tsp salt
freshly ground black pepper
2 tbsp chopped shallots
8 paper-thin lemon slices

In a saucepan over medium heat, cook the plum skins in the chicken stock until the liquid is reduced to 12.5 cl/4 fl oz. Strain the stock and return it to the pan. Reduce the heat to low and add the plum halves and sugar. Simmer the mixture for 1 minute, then remove it from the heat and set aside. Preheat the oven to 190°C (375°F or gas mark 5).

In a shallow, fireproof casserole over medium heat, melt the butter. Lay the breasts in the casserole and sauté them lightly on one side for about 2 minutes. Turn them over, salt and pepper the cooked side, and add the shallots. Place the plum halves, cut side down, between the breasts. Pour the stock into the casserole and arrange two lemon slices on each breast.

Put the uncovered casserole in the oven. Cook until the chicken feels firm but springy to the touch – about 10 minutes. Remove the casserole from the oven and lift out the plums and breasts with a slotted spoon Place them on a warmed platter and return the lemon slices to the sauce. Cover the chicken and plums with foil to keep them warm. Simmer the sauce over medium-high heat until it is reduced to about 4 tablespoons – 5 to 7 minutes. Put the lemon slices back on top of the breasts and arrange the plums around them. Pour the sauce over all and serve.

Honey-basil chicken

4 whole chicken legs, skinned
$1/4$ tsp salt
freshly ground black pepper
1 tbsp safflower oil
7.5 g/$1/4$ oz unsalted butter
2 tbsp honey
2 tbsp unsalted chicken stock
2 garlic cloves, thinly sliced
30 to 40 fresh basil leaves

Preheat the oven to 200°C (400°F or gas mark 6). Cut a piece of aluminium foil 30 cm (1 ft) square for each leg. Sprinkle the legs with the salt and pepper. Heat the oil and butter in a frying pan over medium heat, then brown the legs for about 2 minutes on each side. Put a leg in the middle of each foil square and dribble 1¹/2 teaspoons of honey and 1¹/2 teaspoons of stock over each one. Lay one quarter of the garlic slices on each piece, cover with a loose layer of the basil leaves and wrap the foil snugly over the top. Put the foil packages on a baking sheet and set it in the oven.

After 30 minutes, remove a foil package from the oven and unwrap it carefully to preserve the juices. Test to see if done by piercing the thigh with the tip of a sharp knife: if the juices run clear, it is done. If necessary, return the leg to the oven and bake about 5 minutes more.

To serve, undo each package and transfer the legs to a platter. Remove any garlic or basil that sticks to the foil and put them back on the chicken. Pour the collected juices from the foil packages over the legs.

Red pepper pork with mint

500 g/1 lb pork fillet or loin,
   trimmed of fat and thinly sliced
1 tbsp virgin olive oil
2 sweet red peppers, seeded,
   deribbed and thinly sliced
freshly ground black pepper
500 g/1 lb tomatoes, skinned,
   seeded and chopped
¹/4 tsp salt
2 tbsp finely chopped fresh mint
45 g/1¹/2 oz fromage frais (optional)

Heat the oil in a heavy frying pan; add the red peppers and sauté for 1 minute. Add the pork slices and brown them over high heat. Season with some black pepper, then cover the pan and reduce the heat to low. After 5 minutes, add the tomatoes; continue to cook, covered, for 10 to 15 minutes, or until the meat is tender and the tomato-pepper mixture is well reduced. Season with the salt and some more pepper if required.

Remove the pan from the heat and leave it to cool for 1 minute, then stir in the mint and, if you are using it, the fromage frais. Serve at once.

Pork Char-Shiu

2 pork fillets (about 300 g/10 oz each), thin ends cut off, trimmed of fat

2 tbsp low-sodium soy sauce or shoyu

3 or 4 spring onions, finely chopped

2.5 cm/1 inch piece fresh ginger root, finely chopped

2 garlic cloves, finely chopped

$1/2$ tsp Sichuan pepper

2 star anise

1 tbsp dry sherry

1 tbsp honey

$1^{1}/_{2}$ tsp red wine vinegar

$1/_{2}$ tsp cornflour or potato flour, mixed with 2 tbsp water

mixed salad leaves, washed and dried

Rub the pork with 1 tablespoon of the soy sauce and leave for 20 minutes in a cool place. In a mortar, pound the spring onions, ginger and garlic to a rough paste with the Sichuan pepper and star anise. Mix in the sherry, the remaining soy sauce, half the honey and 1 teaspoon of the vinegar; coat the pork with the paste and leave it to marinate for 2 to 6 hours in the refrigerator, turning it once or twice.

Remove the pork from the refrigerator, pat it dry with paper towels and discard any dry ingredients that are sticking to it. Strain the marinade and reserve. Prepare a glazing syrup by mixing 1 teaspoon of hot water with the remaining honey and vinegar.

Preheat the grill to very hot: place the meat close to the source of heat and brown it on both sides for 3 to 4 minutes. Move the meat to about 10 cm (4 inches) from the heat source and continue to cook for a further 10 minutes, turning a few times and basting constantly with the glazing syrup. Test to see if done with a skewer – the juice that runs out should be almost clear. Cover the cooked fillet loosely with aluminium foil and leave to rest for 5 minutes.

Heat the reserved marinade to a simmer, add the cornflour or potato flour mixture and bring back to simmer. To serve, cut the fillet across the grain into thin slices and place them on a bed of salad leaves. Serve the marinade separately as a dipping sauce.

Turkey crust pizza
1 kg/2 lb white and dark turkey meat, skinned, minced or finely chopped
45 g/1$^1/_2$ oz dry breadcrumbs
1 spring onion, chopped
2 egg whites, lightly beaten
4 drops Tabasco sauce
2 tsp virgin olive oil
$^1/_4$ tsp salt
freshly ground black pepper

2 tbsp white wine
150 g/5 oz grated low-fat mozza-
    rella and Gruyère cheese, com-
    bined

For the pizza sauce

1 tbsp virgin olive oil
90 g/3 oz onion, finely chopped
1 large sweet green or red pepper,
    halved, seeded, deribbed, cut
    into narrow strips
135 g/4$\frac{1}{2}$ oz thinly sliced mush-
    rooms
1 kg/35 oz canned Italian whole
    plum tomatoes
2 large garlic cloves, finely
    chopped
2 tbsp red wine vinegar
2 tsp sugar
1 tbsp chopped fresh basil, or 1 tsp
    dried basil
$\frac{1}{2}$ tsp dried oregano
$\frac{1}{4}$ tsp salt
freshly ground black pepper

To make the sauce, put the oil in a heavy-bottomed saucepan over medium-low heat and cook the onion for 3 minutes, stirring frequently. Add the pepper strips and mushrooms and cook for 2 minutes. Add the rest of the sauce ingredients. Bring to the boil, reduce the heat and simmer gently for 40 minutes, stirring occasionally.

Preheat the oven to 200°C (400°F or gas mark 6). Combine the breadcrumbs, spring onion, egg whites, Tabasco sauce, 1 teaspoon of the oil, and the salt and pepper in a large bowl. Add 12.5 cl (4 fl oz) of the pizza sauce and the white wine. Mix in the minced turkey.

Rub a shallow 25- to 30-cm (10- to 12-inch) round baking dish with the remaining teaspoon of oil. Spread the turkey mixture evenly over the bottom of the dish, pushing it up all round the sides to resemble a crust. Pour half the warm sauce on to the turkey crust. Cover with the grated cheeses. Ladle the remaining sauce over the cheese layer. Sprinkle with freshly ground black pepper. Place the dish on the upper level of the oven and bake for 15 minutes. Remove and let stand for 5 minutes. Cut in wedges and serve immediately.

Fatless sponge

2 eggs
75 g/3 oz caster sugar
75 g/3 oz self-raising flour

Heat the oven to 170°C (350°F or gas mark 4). Break the eggs into a bowl, whisk lightly and add the sugar. Whisk again until thick and creamy. Sieve the flour and fold into the mixture. Pour into a 7-inch (18-cm) cake tin. Bake for about 30 minutes. When it is cooked, slice in half and sandwich together with low-sugar jam, or low-fat yoghurt and sliced fresh fruit, such as pineapple.

Low-fat ice-cream

(makes 900 ml/1^1/$_2$ pints)
1 diabetic jelly, same flavour as
    yoghurt
900 ml/1^1/$_2$ pints low-fat fruit
    yoghurt
1 egg, separated

3 tbsp skimmed milk powder
mixed with 285 ml/^{1}/$_2$ pint water

Mix the jelly crystals with a little water in a heat-proof bowl.
Place over a pan of hot water and stir until dissolved. Leave
to cool slightly, then stir in the yoghurt. Whisk the egg yolk
until pale, then beat into the yoghurt mixture. Beat in the
milk. Pour the mixture into a freezer tray and freeze for about
25 minutes. Remove and beat well. Whisk the egg white until
stiff, then fold into the mixture. Return to the freezer tray
and freeze until firm.

Note: You can make a low-calorie version of any ice-cream
recipe by simply using low-fat yoghurt instead of cream.

Eating Out

Many slimmers find that eating out is a great challenge to their dieting. Whether you are eating out for business or pleasure, there are five main ways to approach the situation:

1 Forget about the diet altogether.

   This may work for those who eat out *rarely*. The occasional over-indulgence should not ruin your slimming as long as the diet is resumed immediately.

2 Stick to your diet rules.

   This is obviously effective – if you have the self-control to do it. If so, congratulations, and carry on.

3 Indulge and balance.

   Indulge on a moderate, planned scale and 'balance' by reducing your calorie intake the day before and the day after the meal. This is effective if it is planned and strictly adhered to. Remember that restaurants often increase the calorie content of food by their methods of preparation, such as frying meat, adding cream to sauces, using oily salad dressings. Take this into account when 'balancing' your calories.

4 Eat a little of everything that you really like.

   This is effective if 'a little' really is only 'a little'.

5 Eat the lowest-calorie choices available.

   This is a useful system. Learn which are the lower-calorie dishes. Remember, as the customer you are entitled to ask the chef to provide plainly cooked versions of meat, fish or vegetables.

Counting Calories

Choose the method that works best for you and try to avoid restaurants that do not cater for your needs. Many restaurant owners are happy to oblige if asked, but many slimmers use eating out as an excuse to over-indulge.

If you have regular business meals, try to frequent a particular establishment that will be more responsive to your needs.

When eating out, don't forget that it is also essential to limit alcohol intake. An aperitif and a glass of wine can make a big dent in your calorie allowance.

Finally, try to regard the occasions and the company as the main pleasures rather than the food.

Parties

Party-time can be danger-time when you are dieting. A bountiful buffet table is designed to tempt you into overeating, and the dishes are often more calorific than they appear. However the tips below will help you survive whether you are giving or going to a party:

- **Do not** starve yourself all day before a party; you will be so hungry that you might binge.

- **Have** a day of light eating the day before and the day after the party.

- **Decide** beforehand whether you will indulge in alcohol, and if so, how much. (Too much alcohol can lead to too much eating.)

- **Make** 'shorts' into long drinks by adding low-calorie mixers. Also add soda water to wine to make a 'spritzer'.

- **Dance** as much as possible; it's enjoyable, uses up calories and minimises time for food and drink.

- **Eat** less of your favourite foods but don't cut them out entirely.

- **Don't** eat something of everything just for the sake of it.
- **Focus** on the company and socialising rather than on the food.

Giving a party?

- **Avoid** serving sausage rolls, vol-au-vents and sausages on sticks; they're boring and very fattening.
- **Serve** visually appealing food, such as tiny rolled-up sandwiches, rolled-up lean meats and colourful rice salads.
- **Offer** low-calorie alternatives wherever possible.
- **Provide** low-calorie dips with fresh vegetable crudités instead of nuts and crisps.
- **Set** aside a plate of carefully chosen low-calorie food for yourself beforehand, then eat no more.
- **Have** low-calorie mixers available, at least for yourself.
- **Put** food and drink in a separate room from the dancing and socialising – it's less tempting.

Going to a party

- **Take** low-calorie mixers with you.
- **Choose** lower-calorie food and don't let yourself feel deprived.
- **Allow** yourself only one serving; leave seconds to others.

Whatever the occasion, enjoy making the most of your slimmer appearance, and remember that you *can* enjoy yourself without overeating.

The demon drink

The words of an old song say, 'Another little drink won't do you any harm', but is this really so?

The wise slimmer is aiming not only to reduce excess weight but also to discover fitness and health.

Of all social habits, drinking alcohol is probably the most difficult to curb. Excess weight is normally associated with food, but alcohol is relatively high in calories and can make big inroads into your daily calorie allowance.

No one denies that alcohol can make you feel good, but it contains no nutrients, so it has no food value. Consequently, it is possible for a heavy drinker to be fat yet still suffer from malnutrition.

Alcohol is sometimes referred to as 'intoxicating liquor', and the word 'toxic' should remind us of its poisonous effects on the body – aggression and violence in the short term, but liver damage, ulcers, high blood pressure, depression, sexual difficulties and brain damage in the long term.

How much is too much?

Recent research by the Health Education Authority indicates that it is safe to drink, provided you keep within recommended guidelines. Alcohol is measured in units, one unit being equal to 250 ml/$^1/_2$ pint ordinary strength beer, or one single pub measure of spirits, sherry, wine or vermouth. The recommended weekly allowance is 21 units for men and 14 units for women (in this instance, female physiology does not allow equality!).

Apart from alcohol's high calorie content, it can have other drawbacks for slimmers. Firstly, it takes effect more quickly because of your reduced food intake; secondly, it impairs judgement, so many a slimmer succumbs to overeating while under the influence; thirdly, the subsequent hangover may lead to consoling yourself with unnecessary food.

If you can, try to exclude alcohol from your diet completely. This may be difficult, especially as alcohol is such a part of the social fabric. However, many people have succeeded in changing their drinking habits, not least because of the impact of 'drink-driving' campaigns.

If you can't give up alcohol, keep your consumption in check and don't be tempted to 'save' your units for a once- or twice-weekly binge. The following tips might help you to reduce your intake.

- 'Home measures' are usually more generous than 'pub measures', so take account of this when calculating your intake.

- 'Low alcohol' does not mean 'low calorie'. Consult a calorie list.

- 'Lengthen' your alcoholic drink by adding soda water or low-calorie mixers.

- Finish one measure of alcohol at a time. Topping up makes it difficult to calculate your intake.

- Pace your alcohol intake throughout an evening and do not get involved in buying rounds.

- Plan alcohol-free days each week and stick to them. This is frequently more successful than making a vague resolve to cut down.

- Say 'no' firmly – not in a way that encourages persuasion.

- If saying no is difficult, take assertion classes or read up about assertion techniques (*see* Further Reading, page 123).

- If you are dependent on alcohol, seek expert advice (*see* Useful Addresses, page 125).

Setting Personal Targets

Target-setting is used successfully in business to improve results. It is based on the principle that if you take time to propose a specific goal and write it down, you are more likely to achieve it than if it remains a vague idea in your mind.

This is also a useful technique for the slimmer because it focuses attention on the weight to be lost in a set period of time. Perhaps, for example, you wish to lose weight for Christmas, a holiday or a special occasion such as a wedding.

- Think ahead. Six weeks is a practical time period.

- Choose the amount of weight you aim to lose in the period. Set realistic targets so you can sustain motivation. Aim to lose an average of 1 kg/2 lb per week, perhaps even a little less. Unrealistic targets simply promote failure and disappointment.

- Weigh yourself at the beginning of your diet and keep a personal record. Each week, reweigh yourself and fill in the details.

- Periodically review your progress towards your target. If you are progressing well, don't use it as an excuse to overindulge. If you are not making much headway, don't despair.

- Review your eating for the week, locate your mistakes and work out how to avoid them next week.

Rewarding Yourself
Many people, especially women, are reluctant to reward themselves. They find it relatively easy to reward others – family,

children and employees – but for various, sometimes complex, reasons they do not extend the same consideration towards themselves. This pattern must be broken if you are to succeed in a long-term task like slimming. In fact, it is essential to build in rewards to sustain your efforts.

Before you jump to conclusions, don't think that rewards necessarily mean food. As children, most of us were given something nice to eat to take away the taste of nasty medicine, to console us after a fall or to congratulate us on passing exams. Consequently, we become conditioned to regard food as reward. This is unhelpful and potentially destructive thinking which the slimmer especially must abandon. How can you do this?

- Stop giving yourself food as a reward. If this is difficult at first, allow yourself 'quality' foods, such as smoked salmon or prawns, rather than the confectionery and sugary treats of your childhood.

- Make a list of the alternatives that could be rewards for you – perhaps a massage or Turkish bath, a professional make-up session, some new clothes, perfume, glossy magazines, coveted records or books. Perhaps you'd like the reward to be spending time by yourself – walking, resting, or even in the bath. Maybe you could make a trip to the theatre or cinema with a friend or organise a babysitter so you can spend extra time alone with your partner.

- Plan your rewards in advance and enjoy anticipating them.

- Mark the successful milestones of your weight-loss, say, each 3 kg/7 lb, with a reward.

Once you've earned your reward, revel in it – you deserve it!

Exercise: Why Bother?

It *is* possible to lose weight without exercising, but slimming is faster and more effective with exercise. Why? Obviously, exercise uses up calories, but it is now thought that there are many extra benefits.

- Metabolism is speeded up – an effect that lasts – so that, after the exercise session, extra calories continue to be used up.
- Muscle develops – the body becomes more shapely.
- A muscle-developed body burns up more calories than a 'flabby' body of the same weight.
- Exercise raises the spirits by causing the brain to release mood-lifting hormones – your own natural antidepressant.
- Physical fitness is enhanced, so you have more energy and stamina.
- Suppleness develops, which makes general movement easier and the body less prone to strains.

What sort of exercise?
Almost any exercise is better than none. For maximum benefit, exercise should be:

- Aerobic
- At least 20 minutes continuously (after warm-up)
- 3–4 times per week

Aerobic exercises always involve having both feet off the ground at some point. They include running, skiing, rowing, cycling, swimming, energetic dancing and brisk walking.

Low-impact aerobic exercise is a fairly new development,

98

designed to minimise injury to joints and muscles. It involves keeping one foot on the ground at all times.

For exercise to be aerobic it must raise the heart rate to within 60–75 per cent of its maximum, as measured by your pulse. Your recommended maximum heart rate can be calculated by subtracting your age from 220 and then calculating 60–75 per cent of that figure.

For example, a person 35 years old would make the following sum:

$220 - 35 = 185$

$185 \times 60\% = 111$

$185 \times 75\% = 139$

- The target zone for this person's pulse rate is between 111 and 139.

- To take your pulse, locate the beat at your wrist with two fingers of one hand. Count the number of beats for 15 seconds. Multiply this number by 4 to obtain the number of beats per minute.

Alternatively, you could buy a pulse-meter, a wristwatch-style device with a monitoring attachment that fastens to a finger or ear. These are available from sports shops.

Starting an exercise programme

Note the following points before you contemplate any kind of exercise:

- Consult your doctor first if you are very unfit, more than 9.5 kg/1½ stones overweight, have any medical condition or are over 40 years old.

- Ease into your exercise programme – too much can be more damaging than too little.

- Start by walking 15 minutes a day, four times a week.

Counting Calories

Table 5: Number of calories burned in 30 minutes of activity (in relation to body weight)

Activity/ exercise	50 kg	55 kg	60kg	65 kg	70 kg	75 kg
Aerobics	155	170	186	200	225	250
Badminton	190	200	210	220	230	240
Basketball	310	350	390	430	470	500
Bowling	95	100	105	110	115	120
Canoeing	120	125	135	140	145	150
Carpentry	125	135	140	145	150	160
Cooking	70	75	80	85	90	95
Cycling	150	165	180	195	210	240
Dancing, moderate	115	120	130	135	140	150
Dancing, fast	300	310	320	330	340	350
Dish-washing	70	75	80	085	90	95
Dressing	40	40	45	45	50	50
Driving	50	55	60	65	70	75
Exercise, moderate	150	160	170	180	190	200
Exercise, fast	200	220	240	260	280	300
Football	275	300	325	350	375	400
Gardening	120	130	140	150	160	170
Golf, no cart	120	125	130	140	145	150
Golf, with cart	70	75	80	85	90	95
Handball	260	275	290	310	330	350
Hockey (field or ice)	300	310	320	330	340	350
Horse-back riding	130	140	150	160	170	180
Housework, active	100	105	110	120	125	135
Ironing	70	70	75	75	80	80
Jogging, light	225	235	245	255	265	275

Activity/ exercise	50 kg	55 kg	60kg	65 kg	70 kg	75 kg
Lacrosse	300	315	330	345	360	375
Office work	65	70	75	80	85	90
Painting (walls)	130	135	140	150	160	170
Piano playing	100	105	110	115	120	125
Reading	15	15	20	20	25	25
Rowing	325	350	375	400	425	450
Running, slow	290	315	345	375	405	435
Running, fast	375	415	450	490	525	550
Sewing	25	25	30	30	35	35
Singing	35	40	45	50	55	60
Sitting at rest	15	15	20	20	25	25
Skating, energetically	250	260	270	280	290	300
Skiing, energetically	250	260	270	280	290	300
Stair climbing	170	185	200	215	230	250
Sweeping floor	70	75	80	90	100	110
Swimming, slow	190	210	230	250	270	290
Swimming, fast	240	260	285	305	330	355
Tennis	165	180	195	215	230	245
Typing	85	90	95	100	105	110
Volleyball	170	185	200	215	230	250
Walking, moderately	105	115	125	135	145	155
Walking, fast	125	135	145	155	165	175
Writing	50	55	60	65	70	75

Increase your speed and time sensibly each week, according to your fitness level.

- Swimming is excellent exercise, whatever your age, and is probably the best choice for those who are very overweight. Join a class if you can't swim. Many pools open early so people can swim before going to work.

- When your fitness level and weight allow, choose other aerobic activities. Walking, running and cycling clubs welcome beginners and the group effort enhances motivation. Alternatively, join an exercise class.

Choosing a class

Whatever kind of exercise class you take, do ensure that it is run by a qualified and experienced teacher who regularly checks your performance. Avoid classes that have too many members to allow proper supervision.

Home exercise

If you prefer to exercise in private, buy an exercise bike and gradually build up to 20-minute sessions. Move through the gears until you are pedalling as hard as possible. To alleviate the boredom of this exercise, read, listen to music or watch television.

Other items of home exercise equipment, such as a rowing machine, mini-trampoline, weights or jogging 'treadmill', can be purchased, if you have enough space and enthusiasm.

Less bulky are the many exercise programmes available on video and audio cassettes. Make sure you do warm-up exercises first and always follow the instructions.

It is all too easy to find excuses for not exercising, especially if you have to juggle work and home commitments. Even if you find it difficult to set time aside for exercise sessions, you can still build activity into your day. For example, use the stairs rather than lifts or escalators, and walk short distances that you usually drive.

The benefits of exercise take a while to show, but your efforts will be rewarded with a fitter, slimmer you.

Physical Aspects of Weight Loss: How the Body Reacts to Dieting

An understanding of the way the body reacts when food intake is restricted is helpful for anyone who is thinking of going on a diet.

The body stores energy in the form of glycogen (animal starch) which is a complex, polysaccharide carbohydrate that is found in liver and muscle cells. If food intake is insufficient to supply the necessary amount of glucose for energy needs, the body turns first to its glycogen stores. Each glycogen molecule incorporates a considerable quantity of water into its structure. This is released by hydrolysis in order to make the glucose part of the molecule available to the body for its shortfall in energy. Water is heavy and during the first week of a diet, three to four pints of it (up to 2.3 litres) are eliminated from the body, as glycogen stores are utilised. This amount of water weighs 3 to 4 lbs (up to 1.8 kg) and accounts for most of the initial 'weight' loss of a diet, but no fat has as yet been eliminated! If you stop the diet after one week, the water (and the weight) is immediately reclaimed as the body replenishes its glycogen stores. It is only as the diet continues that the body begins to utilise its fat stores and this is a much slower process which, as has already been stated, is best achieved at a rate of 1 to 2 lbs (450 to 900 g) per week.

It is important to realise that the body's reaction to a restricted intake of food is to lower the metabolic rate so that fewer calories are required for daily energy needs. This process happens quite quickly and is a physiological survival mechanism, evolved to ensure that life will be prolonged for as long as possible during times of food shortage. Hence, the body reacts to a restricted calorie intake by attempting to conserve its reserves of fat and other tissue. This explains why it can be quite a difficult and slow process to utilise and use up your stores of fat, especially if you are not particularly overweight. Another factor which must be taken into account is that the body utilises muscle and other lean tissue, as well as fat, to provide energy during a diet. This is much more likely to happen if dieting is extreme and so emphasis should be on the importance of adopting a sensible and sustainable approach to losing weight. At the rate of a pound or so a week, loss of lean tissue is minimal and in accordance with the amount of fat being lost. Exercising during dieting helps to preserve muscle and burn up calories and the more lean tissue there is compared to fat, the higher the metabolic rate. Hence exercise can help to counter the natural fall in metabolic rate which accompanies dieting. In general, it will take about three months or so to lose a stone in weight but this varies between different people, according to individual characteristics and the nature of the diet. Once the target weight has been reached and a normal pattern of eating is resumed, the metabolic rate adjusts to its new level. It is normal for a little weight to be regained at the end of the period of dieting but this is water rather than fat and is connected with the body's replenishment of its glycogen stores.

Exercise

There is universal agreement among health experts about the benefits of regular exercise in promoting and maintaining good health and in aiding weight loss during dieting. Exercise helps to relieve various common disorders such as hypertension, depression and constipation and helps to prevent the heart and circulatory diseases that are so prevalent among people in western countries. For all people, even those suffering from certain chronic conditions, exercising within the limits of their strength makes them feel better and promotes restful sleep. The forms and benefits of exercise are discussed in more detail on pages 107 to 108.

Regular physical exercise is vital throughout life to help maintain good health and to confer the ability to remain active, even in old age. Exercise burns up some of the calories in food and so reduces the availability of any excess being laid down as fat. During dieting, exercise uses up a greater proportion of the calories that are consumed so that the body has to turn to its fat stores to provide energy. Fat is naturally deposited and stored in muscle, particularly if muscles are not being properly used. Exercise prevents and reverses this process, increasing the bulk of muscle and using the fat stores as fuel. Muscles are metabolically active even while at rest, so by ensuring that the body has plenty of muscle through regular exercise, more calories are utilised. Exercise confers a sense of well-being, promotes healthy sleep and makes the heart and circulation, lungs and respiration work more efficiently. It also gives you a good appetite, which can be a disadvantage for someone who is dieting and trying to restrict the amount of food being eaten! Vigorous exercise trains the heart so that the muscle fibres become stronger and pump a greater volume of blood with each beat. The result of this is that the resting heartbeat rate slows down and the system works more efficiently. This is achieved by regular, fairly hard activity (called aerobic exercise) which is sufficient to raise the heart and respiration rate for about 15 to 20 minutes, carried out three times each week (or more frequently or for longer, once a person becomes fit). Through its beneficial effects upon the heart and circulation, this type of exercise helps to lower blood pressure, hence reducing the incidence of problems arising from this condition.

Regular exercise training of this sort raises the basal metabolic rate (BMR) which means that the number of calories used while the body is at rest (for respiration, heartbeat, digestion, organ tissue and cell function) is increased. This is one of the great benefits for a dieter since it means that calories from food are more likely to be used and so weight loss is promoted. Non-aerobic 'strength' exercises, particularly some forms of weight-bearing activities, pump calcium into bones and help maintain their density and strength. In older age, this has been shown to significantly reduce the rate at which bone density is lost, hence lessening the risk of fractures.

In summary, different types of exercise and activity can improve bodily health in three main ways:

1 Stamina, fitness or endurance is the ability to sustain a period of vigorous activity without having to stop because your heart is racing and you are gasping for breath! This is built up gradually by an aerobic exercise regime that trains the heart, circulation, lungs and respiration in the manner outlined above. An improvement in fitness is usually noticed quite quickly, after three or four weeks of regular, fairly hard activity and this provides a great encouragement to continue! Unfortunately, however, the level of fitness soon declines if the exercise regime is abandoned, so having worked to make the gains, it is worthwhile to make the effort and find the time to continue. Aerobic exercise, such as vigorous walking, jogging, cycling, dancing, hill walking and many sports – football, tennis, netball, basketball, squash, badminton, etc. – all help to get you fit.

2 Flexibility is the ability of the muscles to perform their full range of movements – twisting, flexing and stretching – with suppleness and ease. There are many exercises that are designed to improve the flexibility and tone of various muscles and joints in different parts of the body and numerous

books and videos are available. For example, many yoga exercises come in to this category. Health practitioners and sports club instructors are normally happy to advise upon the type of exercises that would be of greatest benefit to each individual. Such exercises, which involve stretching, bending and 'loosening up' should always be performed before and after vigorous aerobic activities and sports in order to lessen the risk of injuries or cramps.

3 Strength exercises are aimed at increasing the tone and sometimes the bulk of muscles, leading to the firming up of the body and an improvement in appearance and posture. This reshaping process can, if required, be targeted onto individual trouble spots such as the upper arms, thighs, bottom and stomach. Callanetics, weight training and specially designed gym equipment come into this category but so do a whole series of simple exercises which can be performed at home. Once again, there are many books available on these types of exercises and health and fitness instructors are usually happy to give individual advice. However, anyone who is very unfit or overweight, has an existing medical condition or is aged over 35 is advised to obtain a doctor's advice before attempting to use weights or gym equipment.

Most people recognize the need to undertake physical exercise but for many a perceived lack of free time makes it difficult for them to fit this into their daily routine. People also commonly make the mistake of launching into a fast, vigorous or 'extreme' form of exercise when they are not at all fit to do so. This can be dangerous if there is any underlying, undiagnosed condition such as heart disease or a back or joint problem and may cause illness or injury. In any exercise regime, it is important to be sensible and to increase the level of activity as and when fitness improves. Most vital of all is to stop if it hurts! Contrary to popular belief, pain in exercise is not good for you but is the body's way of telling you that you are doing too much.

People who are prepared to take a critical look at their daily routine usually find that there are slots in their schedule where some physical activity can be fitted in, without causing undue disruption. A well-known and often-quoted example of this is to use the stairs, rather than the lift, at work and to park the car further away in order to fit in a brisk walk or run. It is important to realize that even small measures such as these have a beneficial effect and help to improve fitness, using up some calories and providing a base from which to progress to other forms of exercise. Several routine home activities equally fall into this category including cleaning and vacuuming, decorating and DIY, gardening and mowing the lawn because various muscles are being made to work and the person is actively moving about.

It is advisable for anyone aged over 35 years or who is overweight to check with a doctor before embarking upon a vigorous form of exercise. You should stop if the activity causes discomfort or pain or if you are fighting for breath. Do not exercise hard soon after eating a meal. It is best to eat a starchy meal, which will provide plenty of energy, about three hours before exercising and to drink plenty of water before, during and after the period of activity. You should avoid exercise if you have any form of illness, particularly if you are feverish or anaemic. If you suffer from any form of chronic illness or condition, exercise in accordance with medical advice. Always make sure that you are wearing the correct clothing, footwear and headgear appropriate for the activity and that it is of good quality and fits well. Injuries are often caused through neglect in this area and the cost of equipment is a factor that needs to be taken into account when choosing an exercise or activity.

Finally and most importantly, choose an activity that you enjoy and that is appropriate for you, even if it lies outside the usual range of fitness and exercise regimes. For example, if you enjoy gardening, make this a priority and if your own garden does not present a sufficient challenge how about offering to cut an elderly neighbour's grass? Voluntary and local organisations are always looking for willing, active people to help with a whole range of activities - from maintaining paths to minor (or major!) DIY projects or with helping to set up, and clear up after a fête, fair or show. All this involves active exercise, even if it is different to that being offered by the local health and fitness centre, and usually has the added benefit of being enjoyable from a social pint of view. Certainly, the social aspect of exercise is something else to take into consideration when making a choice of activity – at a dance or karate class or when playing a team sport, you are likely to make new friends.

Although this may seem obvious, people can be influenced by many factors, including what others may say or do and hence do not always make wise choices. Of course, there is no harm in trying a sport or type of exercise to see if you like it, but be prepared to give it up if you do not. The important factor in this case is not to be discouraged but to try something else, rather than thinking that exercise is just not right for you! You are far more likely to succeed in the activity and hence to improve your level of fitness if you enjoy it and look forward to the times when you can carry it out. Dieters have the added bonus of knowing that they are helping themselves to lose weight. Ex-dieters can feel secure in the knowledge that exercising helps the lost pounds to remain that way! But best of all, everyone, whatever their age, weight or shape can be sure that by exercising, they are taking a positive step towards safeguarding their health both for the present and into the future.

The chart on pages 100 and 101 can be used to give you an idea of how many calories (in relation to body weight) you are likely to use when engaged in a variety of activities and exercise.

Overdoing it – a word of warning

Usually, exercise of any sort generates a feeling of wellbeing which is one of the reasons why it is so valuable in the treatment of depression. Hard physical exercise can cause an even more intense experience of elation and exhilaration - an 'exercise high' – which is believed to result from the release of protein substances called endorphins from the pituitary gland at the base of the brain. These are involved in hormonal activity and also have pain-relieving qualities similar to those of morphine. They are released during times of physical stress, as in hard exercise, and it is believed that in these circumstances they cause the feelings of pleasurable exhilaration. Some health experts are concerned that those who regularly exercise hard may be in danger of causing damage to their body in order to achieve this feeling of elation. They may be ignoring warning signs such as pain and may, in some respects, be addicted to the 'exercise high'. Exercising can then become compulsive – something that the person feels that he or she must do, often at the expense of other aspects of life. Compulsive exercising is also a risk factor in eating disorders. If you, or someone you know, comes into this category then it is time to examine what is happening, possibly by talking to a health professional. There is growing evidence that regularly punishing the body with stressful, hard physical exercise is as damaging as not exercising at all. Sudden, unexpected deaths have been reported among those who come into this category and there is increasing concern that these people may suffer damage to organs, skeletal muscle and tendons, which damage which may cause them serious problems in middle and older age.

Troubleshooting

I don't feel like I'm making progress

A combination of balanced diet, aerobic exercise and positive mental attitude are all you need, in theory, to lose weight and be healthy. Why not keep a journal? If at any point you feel you are not progressing as positively as you had hoped then you should be able to go back over your journal and pinpoint where you are going wrong, or whether there has been anything happening in your life that is hindering your progress.

I think I've got a slow metabolism

Remember that those of you who are considerably overweight will be able to lose weight consuming more calories than those of you who are just a little overweight. Contrary to the popular belief that people are fat because of a slow metabolism, actually, fat people have faster metabolisms than those who are naturally slim.

Overweight people, in general, also have more quantities of muscle tissue than slim people. This is because it takes effort and more energy to move around with extra weight. An overweight person will burn more calories than a slim person during identical exercise regimes for how many calories are burned during different activities for people of different weights. On pages 28 to 32 we showed you how to work out your basal metabolic rate. As you lose weight, keep a record of this and your body mass index.

As you lose weight your metabolism may slow down. To contend with this you must ensure that you eat sensibly and exercise so that you do not lose too much lean muscle tissue. Lean muscle tissue is fat-burning tissue. As you lose weight you will feel more energetic and this will help you to progress in your exercise plan. It is normal to gain a little weight after you reach your goal weight and start to eat normally again. Don't be discouraged, just keep putting your new eating habits into practice.

I don't feel like I'm losing weight quickly enough
Most health professionals recommend that you lose 1 to 2 lbs per week. If you combine this with an exercise plan and the use of light weights, this may help to keep the muscles toned and avoid the saggy skin that can sometimes follow weight loss. See pages 98 to 112 for advice on the recommended amount of exercise that you should follow.

Judith Wills, in her book *High Speed Slimming,* insists that there is no hard evidence to show that losing weight quickly is harmful. She argues that it is more encouraging to see quick results, especially in those who are very overweight, than to struggle away for months with little progress. Her book recommends that you exercise a lot to increase the metabolism, eat a healthy, balanced diet in sufficient amounts to maintain your lean muscle tissue and become informed about what you eat. You must never starve yourself. Ask your doctor for his or her advice about such following such a plan. Remember, too much exercise can also be harmful.

Losing weight quickly without re-educating yourself about your diet and without taking care to ask yourself why you eat too much will be disastrous. That is why meal-substitute plans, fad diets and weird food combinations are rarely long-term solutions because it's all too easy to go back to your old habits when you finally crack and can't bear the deprivation any longer.

I'm bored!

If you are bored with a health plan then it may be the wrong one for you.

Why are you bored? Are you eating the same things all the time? Are you following the same exercise plan week after week? Are you exercising on your own? Are you losing weight too slowly?

Write down your favourite healthy foods. Learn new recipes that use them. You don't have to eat broccoli and spinach if you don't like them, but find something equally nutritious that you do enjoy. Do you hate boiled veggies? Spray them with very little garlic-infused olive oil and baste with basamic vinegar and a little honey, sprinkle them with some fresh herbs and sea salt and roast in the oven or barbecue them. Delicious!

If you hate the gym, and a lot of exercise environments are hardly inspiring, why not take a dance class or join a walking group? If your exercise time is more sociable it will be twice as enjoyable.

I'm feel like I'm starving myself

- Eating too little on a diet will create a vicious circle of weight loss and gain.
- Eating too little will make you cranky.
- Eating too little will do you physical harm; you will lose lean muscle tissue and your metabolism will slow down. Your blood sugar will drop and your body will go into starvation mode; it will release levels of potentially damaging adrenaline.
- Eat too little and you are denying yourself the vitamins and essential minerals that keep your skin, hair, and nails looking healthy and attractive.

Counting Calories

If you deny yourself food to the point of starvation you are more likely to binge-eat and feel terrible about yourself afterwards, than if you carefully prepare for yourself a delicious, healthy, balanced meal that actually gives you energy and vitality.

Can I live on fast food?
Low calorie ready-made meals are convenient but are often not very inspiring and sometimes pretty expensive. They are often low in vitamins and fibre and high in highly-processed carbohydrates that are converted by the body into glucose very quickly after they're eaten. Eating processed convenience food like this means that, initially, your blood sugar rises very quickly, your body produces insulin, and then your blood sugar takes a mighty plunge very soon afterwards. High levels of insulin make you want to eat more, and so on.

Here's a little experiment (not recommended for diabetics). For breakfast one morning eat something high in quickly-absorbed carbohydrate (like a Danish pastry, a croissant, or even rice cakes, because although rice cakes are very low-calorie, they have quite a high glycemic index. The glycemic index is a rating system indicating how different foods affect blood sugar. Foods with a low GI are preferable because they are slowly absorbed by the body. Rice cakes have a GI of 82 – that's higher than that of sucrose which is 65! The croissant has a GI of 67. After eating any of these for breakfast, by mid-morning you will be ravenous! Shortly after eating food like this your blood sugar will rise very rapidly and then plummet. If you have porridge, Special K or All Bran and fruit, or some wholegrain rye bread and a scrape of butter instead, then that should keep you going till it's time for lunch because the carbohydrate in these foods is slowly absorbed and this keeps your bood sugar levels stable.

In other words, it's not the number of calories you consume that dictates how full up or hungry you will be, it's the kind of calories. (See *The Glucose Revolution*, Jennie Brand-Miller et al, Hodder Headline, 2000. for the best explanation of this and an excellent comprehensive listing of the glycemic index of foods).

Low-calorie convenience foods and substitutes often don't taste that great. Also, some products imply that they are diet products but are far from it. Food labelled '80% fat free' may sound healthy, but what if they had labelled the product with 'contains 20% fat'? That doesn't sound quite so virtuous. Things that have a diet label on them are not necessarily good for you. If they are low in sugar they may be high in fat or sweeteners. If they are low in fat they may be high in sugar or salt or monosodium glutamate.

It is far, far better to take a real interest in your nutrition and to try to cook interesting, healthy food.

There are plenty of excellent cookery books on the market that will point you in the right direction. There are also lots of sources of low fat recipes on the internet. This book also includes some low fat recipes for you to try.

I hate low-fat food

Most diet plans are low in fat. Everyone agrees that too much fat in the diet is not good for you. Research has also shown, however, that no-fat diets are also bad for you, and some dietitians believe that small amounts of fat eaten at certain times, like a small square of cheese immediately after your main meal, can actually help to curb your appetite.

If you really can't stand the low-calorie substitutes that are available then, for example, use that teaspoonful of olive oil or mayonnaise on your salad if you feel it makes it so much more palatable. Just know when to stop – don't have more than a teaspoon! If you want some chocolate, to the point of not being able to think about anything else, have a *little* chocolate and compensate by cutting down elsewhere and being more active that day. However, if you know that once you get the taste of that chocolate you won't be able stop eating a *lot* of it then I'm afraid you must avoid the demon sweet like the plague and try and distract yourself with something else!

Some foods that are traditionally avoided by dieters are extremely good for us. Nuts are high in fat but are good for us because they are rich in vitamins, minerals and unsaturated fatty acids, so can help to lower cholesterol. Avocado is quite high in fat but is also good for the heart because it contains unsaturated fatty acids, which lower cholesterol, vitamin D and potassium, and has such a low glycemic index that you can count it as zero. It would seem sensible then to eat avocado occasionally and in moderation but not to exclude it entirely from our diets.

I'm counting calories in my sleep!

Try not to get obsessed by calorie counting. Organisations such as Weight Watchers are great if calorie counting bores you and eventually makes you go off your diet. They give you realistic meal and snack ideas. They also give you a bit of moral support to keep you on course and you'll meet people in the same boat as yourself.

Concentrate on good nutrition and sensible food theory (like the glycemic index) and balance your physical activity with the amounts and types of food you eat, so that no food is ever completely banned. Calorie counting is not a waste of time but there are other ways of scrutinising the food we eat, so do take an interest in nutrition.

If you count your calories daily you will eventually be able to judge calorie content approximately just from the weight and ingredients of food. Don't cheat though!

Is fat the only issue?

Do you really need to diet? If you are fit and healthy, and people are always telling you that you don't need to lose weight, could it be that you just need to feel more positive about yourself?

Conversely, if someone is telling you that they think you are too fat, have you thought about your own feelings on the subject? Is this person a positive influence in your life or are they criticising you because of their own inadequacies or out of a need to bring you down to their level?

Do you overeat because you are bored? Maybe you need to find some more interests. Join a group, do a course, plan nights out with friends and try to do something new each time. It could ignite an interest that changes your life.

Do you often think: 'If only I was thinner I would have succeeded'? Some people use being overweight as an excuse when they fail, whether that is in a relationship or a friendship or in their career. Is being fat really the problem?

Be honest, are there other aspects of your life where there are problems but you are too scared, or just not yet able, to deal with them? It is very important that you address these problems whether it be through a counsellor, your doctor or through talking to a close friend.

Do you overeat because you are unhappy? Do you avoid food to punish yourself? If so, then following a diet is never the answer. It is vital that you address your unhappiness by going to a counsellor or by talking to someone close about it. No diet is ever going to solve a problem like this – don't believe in any plan that promises miracles.

- Losing weight should be about improving your life and your health.

- Losing weight is not about trying to look like someone else.

- Losing weight is not about trying to please someone else.
- Losing weight will not necessarily make you more popular.
- Losing weight will not necessarily make you irresistible to the opposite sex.
- Losing weight will not make you more interesting (especially not if you bore your friends with the calorie content of all the foods they eat!)
- Losing weight will not necessarily make you happier.

For the very overweight, losing a lot of weight is sometimes just the first step on their road to good health. Sometimes if one person in a couple accomplishes a huge weight loss the other finds it difficult to adjust to and cope with their partner's new look and new confidence. It can threaten their own role and their security within that relationship.

Remember ...
Eating wonderful food is one of life's seriously great pleasures – but that's the key here, that it is just one of them!

Food should only inhabit a small section of your life, you don't have to think about it all the time. Your family, partner, friends, social life, the friends you are yet to make, work, exercise, hobbies, interests – you need to make room for them all and not place undue importance on your own body image or use food as a crutch when something goes wrong in one of those areas.

Make your dieting as interesting as possible and remember to fit in lots of time for your friends, family and for your interests.

Staying Slim

So, you have reached the ideal/target weight you have set yourself – congratulations!

Now begins the time that many slimmers believe is even more difficult – preventing that excess weight from piling back on.

You have practised new eating habits while on your diet, and now you have lost weight, it is easy to think that you are off the diet and can go back to your old ways of eating. This is a mistake. Your old ways of eating were actually ways of overeating and were the cause of your excess weight.

How to stay slim

- Continue to practise your slim-cooking habits.

- Continue to eat low-fat, no-added-sugar substitutes.

- Continue to 'think slim'.

- Continue to exercise.

- Allow yourself a few extra calories a day, say 100 to begin with, and check that your weight is remaining stable. If not, adjust the extra calories accordingly. You could 'save' the extra calories for a weekend treat.

- Weigh yourself once each week. Don't forget that if you weigh after an indulgent weekend, the extra carbohydrates and sugar will cause some water retention so the weight gain may be more than expected. A stricter weekday routine will soon correct this.

- It may be more realistic to think of staying within a suitable weight range rather than at an exact weight. This allows for premenstrual gains and holiday or seasonal gains.

- As soon as you reach those few pounds above your ideal, apply your slimming principles strictly to reduce the excess.

- Do not crash diet.

- Take note of how your clothes fit. If they start to feel tight, begin your slimming principles immediately – and strictly.

- Don't panic about weight gain. You have learned how to lose weight successfully, so you can do it again, if necessary.

- After the congratulations about your weight loss have died down, you must constantly remind yourself how much better you look and feel in your slim body. Never allow yourself to forget the disadvantages of being overweight, and then you will not allow yourself to slip back into the bad habits that made you fat.

Further Reading

Cookery

Cooking for Your Heart's Content, British Heart Foundation (Arrow, 1978)
The Cook's Handbook, Prue Leith (Macmillan, 1981)
Cooking with Herbs and Spices, Good Housekeeping Institute (Ebury Press, 1975)
Cooking with Herbs and Spices, Jill Graham (Reed, 1984)
The Healthy Gourmet Cookbook, Barbara Bassett (Arlington, 1985)
Low-Fat and No-Fat Cookbook, Jackie Applebee (Thorsons, 1984)
Low-Fat Cookery, Wendy Godfrey (Sainsbury, 1985)
Slim and Fit Family Cookbook, Good Housekeeping Institute (Ebury Press, 1982)
The Slim Gourmet Cookbook, Barbara Gibbons (Harper & Row, 1976)
Slimmers' Microwave Cookbook, Margaret Weale (David & Charles, 1983)
Slimming Menus, Audrey Ellis (Sampson Low, 1979)

Depression and Stress

Beating Depression, Dr John Rush (Century, 1983)
Depression: The Way Out of our Prison, Dorothy Rowe (Routledge & Kegan Paul, 1983)
Stress and Relaxation, Jane Madders (Martin Dunitz, 1980)
Stressmanship, Audrey Livingstone-Booth (Severn House, 1985)

Eating Disorders

Anorexia Nervosa: Let Me Be, A.H. Crisp (Academic Press, 1980)
The Art of Starvation, Sheila Macleod (Virago, 1981)
Bulimarexia, M. Boskind-White and WC. White (Norton, 1983)
Coping with Bulimia, Barbara French (Thorsons, 1987)
Feasting and Fasting, Paulette Maisner (Fontant, 1985)
Hunger Strike, Susie Orbach (Faber, 1986)

Useful Addresses

Eating Disorders

Eating Disorders Association
First Floor
Wensum House
103 Prince of Wales Road
Norwich,
Norfolk,
NR1 1DW,
England
Helpline: 0845 634 1414
   (Mon-Fri 9–6.30)
Youthline: 0845 634 7650
   (Mon–Fri 4–6.30)
Text-phone: 0845 753 322
www.edauk.com

Overeaters Anonymous
Details of support groups
   worldwide.
www.overeatersanonymous.org
info@overeatersanonymous.org

Other relevant websites:
www.caringonline.com
www.anred.com
http://eatingdisorders.
   mentalhelp.net
www.nationaleatingdisorders.org
www.anorectic.fsnet.co.uk

Slimming Organisations

Slimming World
PO Box 55
Alfreton,
Derbyshire, DE55 4U
England
To find a class: 08700 754
   6669
www.slimming-world.co.uk
info@slimming-world.co.uk

Weight Watchers
• UK
Millennium House
Ludlow Road
Maidenhead
Berkshire, SL6 2SL
England
Tel: 08457 123000
www.weightwatchers.co.uk
• USA
www.weightwatchers.com/
   r_vg_index.asp
Tel: 1 800 651 6000
• Canada
www.weightwatchers.com/
   international/canada
• Australia
PO Box 1961

North Sydney, NSW 2059
www.weightwatchers.com.au
New Zealand
www.weightwatchers.co.nz

Counselling and Support
The British Association of
   Counselling
1 Regent Place
Rugby,
Warwickshire,
CV21 2PJ
England
Tel: 0870 443 5252
www.bac.co.uk

Alcoholics Anonymous
•UK
National Helpline: 0845 769
   7555
www.alcoholics-anonymous.
   org.uk
•USA
National Helpline: (212) 870
   3400
Grand Central Station
PO Box 459, New York, NY
   10163
www.alcoholics-anonymous.
   org

The Samaritans
10 The Grove

Slough, Berks, SL1 1QP
England
UK tel: 08457 909090
R of Ireland tel: 1850 609090
www.samaritans.org.uk

National Association for
   Premenstrual Tension
41 Old Road
East Peckham
Kent, TN12 5AP
Tel: 08707 772178
Helpline: 08707 772177

Health and Nutrition
British Association of
   Nutritional Therapists
27 Old Gloucester Road
London,
WC1N 3XX
Tel: 0870 606 1284
www.bant.org.uk
theadministrator@bant.org.uk

Nutrition Society of Australia
PO Box 949
Kent Town,
SA 5071
Australia
Tel: 08 8363 1307
Fax: 08 8363 1604
www.nsa.asn.au
info@nsa.asn.au

The Institute of Optimum
  Nutrition
Blades Court,
Deodar Road
London,
SW15 2LR
Tel: 0208 877 9993
www.ion.ac.uk
info@ion.ac.uk

British Heart Foundation
14 Fitzhardinge Street
London,
W1H 6DH
Tel: 0207 935 0185
ww.bhf.org.uk

Other useful sites:
www.hebs.com
www.nutrition.gov
www.recipeamerica.com
http://nutrition.tufts.edu
www.nutritionaustralia.org
www.intelihealth.com

Diabetes
Diabetes UK Central Office
10 Parkway
London
NW1 7AA
www.diabetes.org.uk
Tel: 020 7424 1030
Text-phone: 020 7424 1888

Nutritional Values

The tables in this book give figures for calories (Kcals) – measurements of the energy value of foods. Calorie-counting is popular as a method of dieting, with the individual following a programme of perhaps 1,500 calories per day or 1,000 calories per day, according to advice.

Figures are also given for carbohydrate, protein and fat content measured in grams. This makes the book useful to those who have chosen, or have been advised to follow, a low-fat or low-carbohydrate diet or who wish to monitor their protein intake.

Fruit

Specific	Amount	Kcals	Carb	Prot	Fat
Apples					
cooking, raw, peeled	100g	35	8.9	0.3	0.1
cooking, stewed with sugar	100g	74	19.1	0.3	0.1
cooking, stewed with sugar	1 portion [140g]	103	26.7	0.4	0.1
cooking, stewed without sugar	100g	33	8.1	0.3	0.1
cooking, stewed without sugar	1 portion [140g]	46	11.3	0.4	0.1
eating, raw, without core	100g	47	11.8	0.4	0.1
eating, raw, with core	100g	42	10.5	0.4	0.1
eating, raw, with core	1 small [75g]	32	7.9	0.3	0.1
eating, raw, with core	1 medium [112g]	47	11.8	0.4	0.1
eating, raw, with core	1 large [170g]	71	17.9	0.7	0.2
eating, raw, peeled	100g	45	11.2	0.4	0.1
Apricots					
canned in juice	100g	34	8.4	0.5	0.1
canned in juice	1 portion [140g]	48	11.8	0.7	0.1
canned in syrup	100g	63	16.1	0.4	0.1
canned in syrup	1 portion [140g]	88	22.5	0.6	0.1
raw, without stone	100g	31	8.5	0.3	0.1
raw, without stone	1 [65g]	20	5.5	0.2	0.1
semi-dried, ready-to-eat	100g	158	36.5	4.0	0.6
Avocado					
raw, without skin or stone	100g	190	1.9	1.9	19.5
raw, without skin or stone	1 small [100g]	190	1.9	1.9	19.5
raw, without skin or stone	1 medium [145]	275	2.8	2.8	28.3
raw, without skin or stone	1 large [195g]	371	3.7	3.7	38.0

Specific	Amount	Kcals	Carb	Prot	Fat
Banana					
with skin	100g	95	23.2	1.2	0.3
with skin	1 small [130g]	123	30.2	1.6	0.4
with skin	1 medium [150g]	143	34.8	1.8	0.5
with skin	1 large [180g]	171	41.8	2.2	0.5
Blackberries	100g	62	15.3	0.8	0.2
stewed with sugar	100g	56	13.8	0.7	0.2
stewed with sugar	1 portion [140g]	78	19.3	1.0	0.3
stewed without sugar	100g	21	4.4	0.8	0.2
stewed withour sugar	1 portion [140g]	29	6.2	1.1	0.3
Blackcurrants	100g	28	6.6	0.9	trace
canned in juice	100g	31	7.6	0.8	trace
canned in syrup	100g	72	18.4	0.7	trace
stewed with sugar	100g	58	15.0	0.7	trace
stewed with sugar	1 portion [140g]	81	21.0	1.0	trace
Cherries					
canned in syrup	100g	71	18.5	0.5	trace
cherries, glace	100g	251	66.4	0.4	trace
raw, without stone	100g	48	11.5	0.9	0.1
raw, without stone	1 [10g]	5	0.6	trace	trace
cherry pie filling	100g	82	21.5	0.4	trace
Clementines					
raw, without skin	100g	37	8.7	0.9	0.1
raw, without skin	1 small [40g]	15	3.5	0.4	trace
raw, without skin	1 medium [60g]	22	5.2	0.5	0.1
raw, without skin	1 large [80g]	30	7.0	0.7	0.1
Currants	100g	267	67.8	2.3	0.4
Damsons					
raw, without stones	100g	34	8.6	0.5	trace
raw, without stones	1 [15g]	5	1.3	trace	trace
stewed with sugar	100g	74	19.3	0.4	trace
stewed with sugar	1 portion [140g]	104	27.0	0.6	trace
Dates					
dried, with stones	100g	227	57.1	2.8	0.2

Calorie Values

Specific	Amount	Kcals	Carb	Prot	Fat
dried, with stone	1 [20g]	45	11.4	0.6	trace
raw, with stones	100g	107	26.9	1.3	0.1
raw, with stone	1 [30g]	32	8.1	0.4	trace
Figs					
dried	100g	227	52.9	3.6	1.6
dried	1 [20g]	45	10.6	0.7	0.3
semi-dried, ready-to-eat	100g	209	48.6	3.3	1.5
semi-dried, ready-to-eat	1 [35g]	73	17.0	1.2	0.5
Fruit pie filling					
average	100g	77	20.1	0.4	trace
Fruit cocktail					
canned in juice	100g	29	7.2	0.4	trace
canned in juice	1 portion [105g]	30	7.6	0.4	trace
canned in syrup	100g	57	14.8	0.4	trace
canned in syrup	1 portion [105g]	60	15.5	0.4	trace
Fruit salad					
home made [bananas, oranges,apples, pears and grapes]	100g	55	13.8	0.7	0.1
home made [bananas, oranges,apples, pears and grapes]	1 portion [140g]	77	19.3	1.0	0.1
Gooseberries	100g	19	3.0	1.1	0.4
dessert, canned in syrup	100g	73	18.5	0.4	0.2
dessert, canned in syrup	1 portion [105g]	77	19.4	0.4	0.2
stewed with sugar	100g	54	12.9	0.7	0.3
stewed with sugar	1 portion [140g]	76	2.7	1.0	0.4
stewed without sugar	100g	16	2.5	0.9	0.3
stewed without sugar	1 portion [140g]	22	3.5	1.3	0.4
Grapefruit					
canned in juice	100g	30	7.3	0.6	trace
canned in juice	1 portion [105g]	32	7.7	0.6	trace
canned in syrup	100g	60	15.5	0.5	trace
canned in syrup	1 portion [105g]	63	16.3	0.5	trace

Specific	Amount	Kcals	Carb	Prot	Fat
raw, with skin	100g	20	4.6	0.5	0.1
raw, with skin	1 small [250g]	50	11.5	1.3	0.3
raw, with skin	1 medium [340g]	68	15.6	1.7	0.3
raw, with skin	1 large [425g]	85	19.6	2.1	0.4
Grapes					
raw, black and white	100g	60	15.4	0.4	0.1
raw, black and white	1 [5g]	3	0.8	trace	trace
Kiwi fruit					
raw, without skin	100g	49	10.6	1.1	0.5
raw, without skin	1 [60g]	29	6.3	0.7	0.3
Lemons					
raw, with peel	100g	19	3.2	1.0	0.3
raw, with peel	1 medium [125g]	24	4.0	1.3	0.3
Lychees					
canned in syrup	100g	68	17.7	0.4	trace
canned in syrup	1 portion [105g]	71	18.6	0.4	trace
raw, without stone	100g	58	14.3	0.9	0.1
raw, without stone	1 [15g]	9	2.1	o.1	trace
Mandarin oranges					
canned in juice	100g	32	7.7	0.7	trace
canned in juice	1 portion [105g]	34	8.1	0.7	trace
canned in syrup	100g	52	13.4	0.5	trace
canned in syrup	1 portion [105g]	55	14.1	0.5	trace
Mangoes					
canned in syrup	100g	77	20.3	0.3	trace
canned in syrup	1 portion [105g]	81	21.3	0.3	trace
raw, without stone or skin	100g	57	14.1	0.7	0.2
raw, without stone or skin	1 slice [40g]	23	5.6	0.3	trace
Melon					
Canteloupe, without skin or seeds	100g	19	4.2	0.6	0.1
Canteloupe, without skin or seeds	1 slice [150g]	29	6.3	0.9	0.2
Galia, without skin or seeds	100g	24	5.6	0.5	0.1

Calorie Values

Specific	Amount	Kcals	Carb	Prot	Fat
Galia, without skin or seeds	1 slice [150g]	36	8.4	0.8	0.2
Honeydew, without skin or seeds	100g	28	6.6	0.6	0.1
Honeydew, without skin or seeds	1 slice [180g]	50	11.8	1.1	0.2
Watermelon, without skin or seeds	100g	31	7.1	0.5	0.3
Watermelon, without skin or seeds	1 slice [200g]	62	14.2	1.0	0.6
Mixed fruit					
dried	100g	268	68.1	2.3	0.4
dried	1 tbsp [25g]	67	17.0	0.6	0.1
Nectarines					
raw, without stones	100g	40	9.0	1.4	0.1
raw, without stone	1 small [125g]	50	11.3	1.8	0.1
raw, without stone	1 medium [140g]	56	12.6	2.0	0.1
raw, without stone	1 large [175g]	70	15.8	3.5	0.2
Olives					
in brine	100g	103	trace	0.9	11.0
in brine	1 [3g]	3	trace	trace	0.3
Oranges					
raw, without skin	100g	37	8.5	1.1	0.1
raw, without skin.	1 small [120g]	46	10.6	1.4	0.1
raw, without skin	1 medium [160g]	59	13.6	2.2	0.2
raw, without skin	1 large [210g]	78	17.9	2.3	2.2
Passion fruit					
raw, without skin	100g	36	5.8	2.6	0.4
raw, without skin	1 [15g]	5	0.9	0.4	trace
Paw-paw					
raw	100g	36	8.8	0.5	0.1
Peaches					
canned in juice	100g	39	9.7	0.6	trace
canned in juice	1 portion [105g]	41	10.2	0.6	trace

Specific	Amount	Kcals	Carb	Prot	Fat
canned in syrup	100g	55	14.0	0.5	trace
canned in syrup	1 portion [105g]	58	14.7	0.5	trace
raw, without stone	100g	33	7.6	1.0	0.1
raw, without stone	1 small [70g]	23	5.3	0.7	trace
raw, without stone	1 medium [110g]	36	8.4	1.1	0.1
raw, without stone	1 large [150g]	50	11.4	1.5	0.2
Pears					
canned in juice	100g	33	8.5	0.3	trace
canned in juice	1 portion [120g]	40	10.2	0.4	trace
canned in syrup	100g	50	13.2	0.2	trace
canned in syrup	1 portion [120g]	60	15.8	0.2	trace
raw, without core	100g	40	10.0	0.3	0.1
raw, without core	1 medium [200g]	80	20.0	0.6	0.2
raw, peeled	100g	41	10.4	0.3	0.1
Peel					
mixed, dried	100g	231	59.1	0.3	0.9
Pineapple					
canned in juice	100g	47	12.2	0.3	trace
canned in juice	1 portion [120g]	56	14.6	0.3	trace
canned in syrup	100g	64	16.5	0.5	trace
canned in syrup	1 portion [120g]	77	20	0.6	trace
raw, without skin	100g	41	10.1	0.4	0.2
raw, without skin	1 slice [80g]	33	8.1	0.3	0.2
Plums					
canned in syrup	100g	59	15.5	0.3	trace
canned in syrup	1 portion [105g]	62	16.3	0.3	trace
raw, without stone	100g	34	8.3	0.5	0.1
raw, without stone	1 small [30g]	10	2.5	0.2	trace
raw, without stone	1 medium [55g]	19	4.6	0.3	0.1
raw, without stone	1 large [85g]	29	7.1	0.4	0.1
stewed with sugar, weighed with stones	100g	75	19.2	0.5	0.1
stewed with sugar, weighed with stones	1 portion [140g]	105	26.9	0.7	0.1

Calorie Values

Specific	Amount	Kcals	Carb	Prot	Fat
stewed without sugar, weighed with stones	100g	29	6.9	0.4	0.1
stewed without sugar, weighed without stones	1 portion [140g]	41	9.7	0.6	0.1
Prunes					
canned in juice	100g	79	19.7	0.7	0.2
canned in juice	1 portion [105g]	83	20.7	0.7	0.2
canned in syrup	100g	90	23.0	0.6	0.2
canned in syrup	1 portion [105g]	95	24.2	0.6	0.2
semi-dried, ready-to-eat	100g	141	34.0	2.5	0.4
semi-dried, ready-to-eat	1 [15g]	21	5.1	0.4	trace
Raisins	100g	272	69.3	2.1	0.4
	1 tbsp [30g]	82	20.8	0.6	trace
Raspberries					
canned in syrup	100g	31	7.6	0.5	trace
canned in syrup	1 portion [105g]	33	8.0	0.5	trace
raw	100g	25	4.6	1.4	0.3
raw	1 portion [60g]	15	2.8	0.8	0.2
Rhubarb					
canned in syrup	100g	65	16.9	0.5	trace
canned in syrup	1 portion [140g]	91	23.7	0.7	trace
raw	100g	7	0.8	0.9	0.1
stewed with sugar	100g	48	11.5	0.9	0.1
stewed with sugar	1 portion [140g]	67	16.1	1.3	0.1
stewed without sugar	100g	7	0.7	0.9	0.1
stewed without sugar	1 portion [140g]	10	1.0	1.3	0.1
Satsumas					
raw, without peel	100g	36	8.5	0.9	0.1
raw, without peel	1 small [50g]	18	4.3	0.5	0.1
raw, without peel	1 medium [70g]	25	6.0	0.6	0.1
raw, without peel	1 large [90g]	32	7.7	0.8	0.1
Strawberries					
canned in syrup	100g	65	16.9	0.5	trace
canned in syrup	1 portion [105g]	68	17.9	0.5	trace

Specific	Amount	Kcals	Carb	Prot	Fat
raw	100g	27	6.0	0.8	0.1
raw	.1 [12g]	3	6.1	0.1	trace
Sultanas	100g	275	69.4	2.7	0.4
	1 tbsp [30g]	83	20.8	0.8	trace
Tangerines					
raw	100g	35	8.0	0.9	0.1
raw	1 small [50g]	18	4.0	0.5	0.1
raw	1 medium [70g]	25	5.6	0.6	0.1
raw	1 large [90g]	32	7.2	0.6	0.1

Vegetables

Specific	Amount	Kcals	Carb	Prot	Fat
Asparagus					
boiled	100 g	26	1.4	3.4	0.8
boiled	1 portion[125g/ approx 5 spears]	33	1.7	4.3	1.0
raw	100g	25	2.0	2.9	0.6
Aubergine					
fried in corn oil	100g	302	2.8	1.2	31.9
fried in corn oil	1 portion [130g]	393	3.6	1.6	41.5
raw	100g	15	2.2	0.9	0.4
Bamboo Shoots					
canned, drained	100g	39	9.7	0.7	0
canned, drained	225g can	88	21.8	1.6	0
Beans					
Aduki, dried, boiled	100g	123	22.5	9.3	0.2
Aduki, dried, boiled	1 tbsp [30g]	37	6.8	2.8	trace
Baked, canned in tomato sauce	100g	84	15.3	5.2	0.6
Baked, canned in tomato sauce	1 small portion [80g]	67	12.2	4.2	0.5
Baked, canned in tomato sauce	1 medium portion [135g]	113	20.7	7.0	0.8
Baked, canned in tomato sauce	1 large portion [190g]	160	29.1	9.9	1.1
Baked, canned in tomato sauce	1 tbsp [45g]	38	6.9	2.3	0.3
Baked, canned in tomato sauce, reduced sugar	100g	73	12.5	5.4	0.6
Baked, canned in tomato sauce, reduced sugar	1 small portion [80g]	58	10.0	4.3	0.5

136

Specific	Amount	Kcals	Carb	Prot	Fat
Baked, canned in tomato sauce, reduced sugar	1 medium portion [135g]	99	16.9	7.3	0.8
Baked, canned in tomato sauce, reduced sugar	1 large portion [190g]	139	23.8	10.3	1.1
Baked, canned in tomato sauce, reduced sugar	1 tbsp [45g]	33	5.6	2.4	0.3
Blackeye, dried, boiled	100g	116	19.9	8.8	0.7
Blackeye, dried, boiled	1 tbsp [45g]	52	8.9	3.9	0.3
Broad, frozen, boiled	100g	81	11.7	7.9	0.6
Broad, frozen, boiled	1 portion [120g]	96	14.0	9.5	0.7
Butter, canned, re-heated, drained	100g	77	13.0	5.9	0.5
Butter, canned, re-heated, drained	1 portion [120g]	92	15.6	7.1	0.6
French, frozen, boiled	100g	25	4.7	1.7	0.1
French, frozen, boiled	1 small portion [60g]	15	2.8	1.0	0.1
French, frozen, boiled	1 medium portion [90g]	23	4.2	1.5	0.1
French, frozen, boiled	1 large portion [120g]	30	5.6	2.0	0.1
French, raw	100g	24	3.2	1.9	0.5
Mung, dried, boiled	100g	91	15.3	7.6	0.4
Mung, dried, boiled	1 tbsp [30g]	27	4.6	2.3	0.1
Red kidney, canned, re-heated, drained	100g	100	17.8	6.9	0.6
Red kidney, canned, re-heated, drained	1 portion [120g]	120	21.4	8.3	0.7
Red kidney, dried, boiled	100g	103	17.4	8.4	0.5
Red kidney, dried, boiled	1 tbsp [30g]	31	5.2	2.5	0.2
Runner, boiled	100g	186	2.3	1.2	0.5
Runner, boiled	60g portion	11	1.4	0.7	0.2
Runner, boiled	90g portion	16	2.1	1.1	0.5
Runner, boiled	120g portion	22	2.8	1.4	0.6

Calorie Values

Specific	Amount	Kcals	Carb	Prot	Fat
Runner, raw	100g	22	3.2	1.6	0.4
Soya, dried, boiled	100g	141	5.1	14.0	7.3
Soya, dried, boiled	1 tbsp [30g]	42	1.5	4.2	2.2
Beansprouts					
Mung, stir-fried in oil	100g	72	2.5	1.9	6.1
Mung, stir-fried in oil	1 portion [90g]	65	2.3	1.7	5.5
Mung, raw	100g	31	4.0	2.9	0.5
Beetroot					
boiled	100g	46	9.5	2.3	0.1
boiled	1 slice [10g]	5	1.0	0.2	trace
pickled, drained	100g	28	5.6	1.2	0.2
pickled, drained	1 slice [10g]	3	0.6	0.1	trace
raw	100g	36	7.6	1.7	0.1
Black gram					
dried, boiled	100g	89	13.6	7.8	0.4
Broccoli					
boiled	100g	24	1.1	3.1	0.8
boiled	1 portion [90g]	22	1.0	2.8	0.7
raw	100g	33	1.8	4.4	0.9
Brussels sprouts					
boiled	100g	35	3.5	2.9	1.3
boiled	1 small portion [60g]	21	2.1	1.7	0.8
boiled	1 medium portion [90g]	32	3.2	2.6	1.2
boiled	1 large portion [120g]	42	4.2	3.5	1.6
frozen, boiled	100g	35	2.5	3.5	1.3
frozen, boiled	1 small portion [60g]	21	1.5	2.1	0.8
frozen, boiled	1 medium portion [90g]	32	2.3	3.2	1.2
frozen, boiled	1 large portion [120g]	42	3.0	4.2	1.6

138

Specific	Amount	Kcals	Carb	Prot	Fat
raw	100g	42	4.1	5.3	1.4
Cabbage					
boiled	100g	18	2.5	0.8	0.6
boiled	1 small				
	portion [60g]	11	1.5	0.5	0.4
boiled	1 medium				
	portion [90g]	16	2.3	0.7	0.4
boiled	1 large				
	portion [120g]	22	3.0	1.0	0.4
raw	100g	26	4.1	1.7	0.4
raw	1 medium				
	portion [90g]	23	3.7	1.5	0.4
white, raw	100g	27	5.0	1.4	0.2
white, raw	1 medium				
	portion [90g]	24	4.5	1.3	0.2
Carrots					
canned, re-heated, drained	100g	20	4.2	0.5	0.3
canned, re-heated, drained	3 carrots [35g]	7	1.5	0.2	0.1
old, boiled	100g	24	4.9	0.6	0.4
old, boiled	1 small				
	portion [40g]	10	2.9	0.4	0.2
old, boiled	1 medium				
	portion [60g]	14	1.2	0.2	0.1
old, boiled	1 large				
	portion [85g]	20	1.7	0.2	0.1
old, raw	100g	35	2.5	0.3	0.2
old, raw	1 medium				
	portion [60g]	21	1.5	0.2	0.1
young, boiled	100g	22	4.4	0.6	0.4
young, boiled	1 medium				
	portion [60g]	13	2.6	0.4	0.2
young, raw	100g	30	6.0	0.7	0.5

Calorie Values

Specific	Amount	Kcals	Carb	Prot	Fat
young, raw	1 medium portion [60g]	18	3.6	0.4	0.3
Cauliflower					
boiled	100g	28	2.1	2.9	0.9
boiled	1 small portion [60g]	17	1.3	1.7	0.5
boiled	1 medium portion [90g]	25	1.9	2.6	0.8
boiled	1 large portion [120g]	34	2.5	3.5	1.1
raw	100g	34	3.0	3.6	0.9
raw	1 floret [10g]	3	0.3	0.4	trace
Celery					
boiled	100g	8	0.8	0.5	0.3
boiled	1 small portion [30g]	2	0.2	0.2	0.1
boiled	1 medium portion [50g]	4	0.4	0.3	0.2
boiled	1 large portion [85g]	7	0.7	0.4	0.3
raw	100g	7	0.9	0.5	0.2
raw	1 stick [30g]	2	0.3	0.2	0.1
Chick peas					
canned, re-heated, drained	100g	115	16.1	7.2	2.9
canned, re-heated, drained	1 medium portion [90g]	104	14.5	6.5	2.6
dried, boiled	100g	121	18.2	8.4	2.1
dried, boiled	1 heaped tbsp [28g]	34	5.1	2.4	0.6
Chicory					
raw	100g	11	2.8	0.5	0.6
Courgette					
boiled	100g	19	2.0	2.0	0.4

Specific	Amount	Kcals	Carb	Prot	Fat
boiled	1 small portion [60g]	11	1.2	1.2	0.2
boiled	1 medium portion [90g]	17	1.8	1.8	0.2
boiled	1 large portion [120g]	23	2.4	2.4	0.2
fried in corn oil	100g	63	2.6	2.6	4.8
fried in corn oil	1 small portion [60g]	38	1.6	1.6	2.9
fried in corn oil	1 medium portion [90g]	57	2.3	2.3	4.3
fried in corn oil	1 large portion [120g]	76	3.1	3.1	5.8
raw	100g	18	1.8	1.8	0.4
Cucumber					
raw	100g	10	1.5	0.7	0.1
raw	1-inch piece [60g]	6	0.9	0.4	0.1
Curly Kale					
boiled	100g	24	1.0	2.4	1.1
boiled	1 medium portion [90g]	14	0.6	1.4	0.7
raw	100g	33	1.4	3.4	1.6
Fennel					
boiled	100g	11	1.5	0.9	0.2
boiled	1 medium portion [50g]	6	0.8	0.5	0.1
raw	100g	12	1.8	0.9	0.2
Garlic					
raw	100g	98	16.3	7.9	0.6
Gherkins					
pickled, drained	100g	14	2.6	0.9	0.1
Gourd					
raw	100g	11	0.8	1.6	0.2

Calorie Values

Specific	Amount	Kcals	Carb	Prot	Fat
Hummus	100g	187	11.6	7.6	12.6
	1 tbsp [50g]	94	5.8	3.8	6.3
Leeks					
boiled	100g	21	2.6	1.2	0.7
boiled	1, average size [160g]	34	4.2	1.9	1.1
raw	100g	22	2.9	1.6	0.5
Lentils					
green and brown, whole, dried, boiled	100g	105	16.9	8.8	0.7
green and brown, whole, boiled	1 tbsp [30g]	32	5.1	2.6	0.2
red, split, dried, boiled	100g	100	17.5	7.6	0.4
red, split, dried, boiled	1 tbsp [30g]	30	5.3	2.3	0.1
Lettuce					
average, raw	100g	14	1.7	0.8	0.5
average, raw	1 salad serving [30g]	4	0.5	0.2	0.2
Iceberg, raw	100g	13	1.9	0.7	0.3
Iceberg, raw	1 salad serving [80g]	10	0.6	0.2	0.1
Marrow					
boiled	100g	9	1.6	0.4	0.2
raw	100g	12	2.2	0.5	0.2
Mixed vegetables					
frozen, boiled	100g	42	6.6	3.3	0.5
frozen, boiled	1 medium serving [90g]	38	5.9	3.0	0.5
with chilli, canned	100g	86	9.1	4.3	3.8
with chilli, canned	400g can	345	36.0	17.0	15.0
Mushrooms					
boiled	100g	11	0.4	1.8	0.3
creamed, canned	100g	80	5.4	3.4	5.0
creamed, canned	210g can	168	11.3	7.1	10.5

Specific	Amount	Kcals	Carb	Prot	Fat
fried in blended oil	100g	157	0.3	2.4	16.2
fried in butter	100g	157	0.3	2.4	16.2
fried in corn oil	100g	157	0.3	2.4	16.2
fried	1 medium portion [45g]	71	0.1	1.1	7.3
raw	100g	135	0.4	1.8	0.5
raw	1, average [10g]	1	trace	0.2	trace
Mustard and Cress					
raw	100g	13	0.4	1.6	0.6
raw	1 tbsp [5g]	1	trace	0.1	trace
raw	1 punnet [40g]	5	0.2	0.6	0.2
Okra					
boiled	100g	28	2.7	2.5	0.9
raw	100g	31	3.0	2.8	1.0
raw	10, medium [50g]	16	1.5	1.4	0.5
stir-fried in corn oil	100g	269	4.4	4.3	26.1
stir-fried in corn oil	1 medium portion [60g]	161	2.6	2.6	15.7
Onions					
boiled	100g	17	3.7	0.6	0.1
boiled	1 medium portion [60g]	10	2.2	0.4	0.1
cocktail/ silverskin, drained	100g	15	3.1	0.6	0.1
fried in blended oil	100g	164	14.1	2.3	11.2
fried in corn oil	100g	164	14.1	2.3	11.2
fried in lard	100g	164	14.1	2.3	11.2
fried	1 medium portion [57g]	98	8.5	1.4	6.7
pickled, drained	100g	24	4.9	0.9	0.2
pickled, drained	1, average [10g]	2	0.5	0.1	trace
pickled, drained	1, large [25g]	6	1.2	0.2	trace
raw	100g	36	7.9	1.2	0.2
raw	1, average [90g]	32	7.1	1.1	0.2

Calorie Values

Specific	Amount	Kcals	Carb	Prot	Fat
raw	1 slice [20g]	7	1.6	0.2	trace
Parsnip					
boiled	100g	66	12.9	1.6	1.2
boiled	1 small portion [40g]	26	5.2	0.6	0.5
boiled	1 medium portion [65g]	43	8.4	1.0	0.7
boiled	1 large portion [85g]	56	11.0	1.4	1.0
raw	100g	64	12.5	1.8	1.1
Peas					
boiled	100g	79	10.0	6.7	1.6
boiled	1 small portion [40g]	32	4	2.7	0.6
boiled	1 medium portion [65g]	51	6.5	4.4	1.0
boiled	1 large portion [85g]	67	8.5	5.7	1.4
canned, re-heated, drained	100g	80	13.5	5.3	0.9
canned, re-heated, drained	1 tbsp [30g]	24	4.1	1.6	0.3
frozen, boiled	100g	69	9.7	6.0	0.9
frozen, boiled	1 medium portion [65g]	45	6.3	3.9	0.6
Mange-tout, boiled	100g	261	3.3	3.2	0.1
Mange-tout, boiled	1 medium portion [50g]	13	1.7	1.6	0.1
Mange-tout, raw	100g	32	4.2	3.6	0.2
Mange-tout, stir-fried in blended oil	100g	71	3.5	3.8	4.8
mushy, canned, re-heated, drained	100g	81	13.8	5.8	0.7
mushy, canned,					

Specific	Amount	Kcals	Carb	Prot	Fat
re-heated, drained	1 tbsp [30g]	24	4.1	1.7	0.2
Petits pois, frozen, boiled	100g	49	5.5	5.0	0.9
Petits pois, frozen, boiled	1 medium portion [65g]	32	3.6	3.3	0.6
processed, canned, re-heated, drained	100g	99	17.5	6.9	0.7
processed, canned, re-heated, drained	1 tbsp [30g]	30	5.3	2.1	0.2
raw	100g	83	11.3	6.9	1.5
Peppers					
Capsicum, green, boiled	100g	18	2.6	1.0	0.5
Capsicum, green, raw	100g	15	2.6	0.8	0.3
Capsicum, green, raw	1, medium [160g]	24	4.2	1.3	0.5
Capsicum, green, raw	1 sliced ring [10g]	2	0.3	0.1	trace
Capsicum, red, boiled	100g	34	7.0	1.1	0.4
Capsicum, red, raw	100g	32	6.4	1.0	0.4
Capsicum, red, raw	1, medium [160g]	51	10.2	1.6	0.6
Capsicum, red, raw	1 sliced ring [10g]	3	0.6	0.1	trace
mixed, raw	100g	20	0.7	2.9	0.6
Plantain					
boiled	100g	112	28.5	0.8	0.2
boiled	1, whole [200g]	224	57.0	1.6	0.4
fried in vegetable oil	100g	267	47.5	1.5	9.2
raw	100g	117	29.4	1.1	0.3
Potato croquettes					
fried in blended oil	100g	214	21.6	3.7	13.1
fried in blended oil	1, average [80g]	171	17.3	3.0	0.9
Potato powder					
instant, made up with water	100g	57	13.5	1.5	0.1

Calorie Values

Specific	Amount	Kcals	Carb	Prot	Fat
instant, made up with water	1 medium portion [180g]	103	24.3	2.7	0.18
instant, made up with whole milk	100g	76	14.8	2.4	1.2
instant, made up with whole milk	1 medium portion [180g]	137	26.7	4.3	2.2
Potato waffles	100g	842	30.3	3.2	8.2
Potatoes (Chips)					
fine cut, frozen, fried in blended oil	100g	364	41.2	4.5	21.3
fine cut, frozen, fried in corn oil	100g	364	41.2	4.5	21.3
fine cut, frozen, fried in dripping	100g	364	41.2	4.5	21.3
fine cut, frozen, fried	1 small portion [130g]	473	53.6	5.9	27.7
fine cut, fried	1 medium portion [180g]	655	74.2	8.1	38.3
fine cut, fried	1 large portion [240g]	874	98.9	10.8	51.12
homemade, fried in oil	100g	189	30.1	3.9	6.7
homemade, fried in dripping	100g	189	30.1	3.9	6.7
homemade, fried	1 small portion [130g]	246	39.1	5.1	8.7
homemade, fried	1 medium portion [180g]	340	54.2	7.0	12.1
homemade, fried	1 large portion [240g]	454	72.2	9.4	20.1
oven, frozen, baked	100g	162	29.8	3.2	4.2
oven, frozen, baked	1 medium portion [180g]	292	53.6	5.8	7.6
chip shop, fried in dripping	100g	239	30.5	3.2	12.4

Specific	Amount	Kcals	Carb	Prot	Fat
chip shop, fried in blended oil	100g	239	30.5	3.2	12.4
chip shop, fried in vegetable oil	100g	239	30.5	3.2	12.4
chip shop, fried	1 average serving [200g]	478	61.0	6.4	24.8
straight cut, frozen, fried in blended oil	100g	273	36.0	4.1	13.5
straight cut, frozen, fried in corn oil	100g	273	36.0	4.1	13.5
straight cut, frozen, fried in dripping	100g	273	36.0	4.1	13.5
straight cut, frozen, fried	1 portion [180g]	491	64.8	7.4	24
french fries, retail [burger restaurants]	100g	280	34.0	3.3	15.5
french fries, retail [burger restaurants]	1 regular serving [105g]	294	35.7	3.5	16.3
french fries, retail [burger restaurants]	1 regular serving [150g]	420	51	5.0	23.3
Potatoes (New)					
boiled	100g	75	17.8	1.5	0.3
boiled	1 small portion [120g]	90	21.4	1.8	0.4
boiled	1 medium portion [180g]	135	32.0	2.7	0.5
boiled	1 large portion [220g]	165	39.2	3.3	0.7
boiled in skins	100g	66	15.4	1.4	0.3
boiled in skins	1 small portion [120g]	79	18.5	1.7	0.4
boiled in skins	1 medium portion [180g]	119	27.7	2.5	0.5

Calorie Values

Specific	Amount	Kcals	Carb	Prot	Fat
boiled in skins	1 large portion [220g]	145	33.9	3.1	0.7
canned, re-heated, drained	100g	63	15.1	1.5	0.1
canned, re-heated drained	1 medium portion [180g]	113	27.2	2.7	0.2
raw	100g	70	16.1	1.7	0.3
Potatoes (old)					
baked, flesh and skin	100g	136	31.7	3.9	0.2
baked, flesh and skin	1 medium-size [180g]	245	57.1	7.0	0.4
baked, flesh only	100g	77	18.0	2.2	0.1
baked, flesh only	1 medium-size [160g]	123	28.8	3.5	0.2
boiled	100g	72	17.0	1.8	0.1
boiled	1 small portion [120g]	86	20.4	2.2	0.1
boiled	1 medium portion [180g]	130	30.6	3.2	0.2
boiled	1 large portion [220g]	158	37.4	4.0	0.2
boiled, mashed with butter or margarine	100g	104	15.5	1.8	4.3
boiled, mashed with butter or margarine	1 medium portion [180g]	187	27.9	3.2	7.7
raw	100g	75	17.2	2.1	0.2
roast in blended oil	100g	149	25.9	2.9	4.5
roast in corn oil	100g	149	25.9	2.9	4.5
roast in lard	100g	149	25.9	2.9	4.5
roast	1 medium portion [200g]	298	51.8	5.8	9.0
Pumpkin					
raw	100g	13	2.2	0.7	0.2
boiled	100g	13	2.1	0.6	0.3

Specific	Amount	Kcals	Carb	Prot	Fat
Quorn	100g	86	2.0	11.8	3.5
Radish					
raw	100g	12	1.9	0.7	0.2
raw	1, average [10g]	1	0.2	0.1	trace
Ratatouille					
canned	100g	38	3.0	1.0	2.5
canned	400g can	150	12.0	4.0	10.0
Spinach					
boiled	100g	19	0.8	2.2	0.8
boiled	1 medium portion [90g]	17	0.7	2.0	0.7
frozen, boiled	100g	21	0.5	3.1	0.8
frozen, boiled	1 medium portion [90g]	19	0.5	2.8	0.7
raw	100g	25	1.6	2.8	0.8
Spring greens					
boiled	100g	20	1.6	1.9	0.7
boiled	1 medium portion [90g]	18	1.4	1.7	0.6
raw	100g	33	3.1	3.0	1.0
Spring onions					
raw	100g	23	3.0	2.0	0.5
raw	1, average [20g]	5	0.6	0.4	0.1
Swede					
raw	100g	24	5.0	0.7	0.3
boiled	100g	11	2.3	0.3	0.1
boiled	1 small portion [40g]	4	0.9	0.1	trace
boiled	1 medium portion [60g]	7	1.4	0.1	0.1
boiled	1 large portion [85g]	9	2.0	0.3	0.1
Sweet potato					
boiled	100g	84	20.5	1.1	0.3

Specific	Amount	Kcals	Carb	Prot	Fat
boiled	2, medium [130g]	109	26.7	1.4	0.4
raw	100g	87	21.3	1.2	0.3
Sweetcorn					
baby, canned, drained	100g	23	2.0	2.9	0.4
kernels, canned, drained	100g	122	26.6	2.9	1.2
kernels, canned, drained	1 tbsp [30g]	37	8.0	0.9	0.4
on-the-cob, whole, boiled	100g	66	11.6	2.5	1.4
on-the-cob, whole, boiled	1, kernels only [125g]	83	14.5	3.1	1.8
Tofu					
Soya bean, steamed	100g	73	0.7	8.1	4.2
Soya bean, steamed, fried	100g	261	2.0	23.5	17.7
Tomatoes and tomato-based products					
canned, with juice	100g	16	3.0	1.0	0.1
fried in blended oil	100g	91	5.0	0.7	7.7
fried in corn oil	100g	91	5.0	0.7	7.7
fried in lard	100g	91	5.0	0.7	7.7
grilled	100g	49	8.9	2.0	0.9
Passata	100g	29	6.0	1.1	0.2
Passata	550g jar	160	33.0	6.1	1.1
raw	100g	17	3.1	0.7	0.3
raw	1, small [65g]	11	2.0	0.5	0.2
raw	1, medium [85g]	14	2.6	0.6	0.3
raw	1, large [150g]	26	4.7	0.8	0.3
tomato purée	100g	68	12.9	4.5	0.2
Turnip					
boiled	100g	12	2.0	0.6	0.2
boiled	1 small portion [40g]	5	0.8	0.2	0.1
boiled	1 medium portion [60g]	7	1.2	0.4	0.1

Specific	Amount	Kcals	Carb	Prot	Fat
boiled	1 large portion [85g]	10	1.7	0.5	0.2
raw	100g	23	4.7	0.9	0.3
Watercress					
raw	100g	22	0.4	3.0	1.0
raw	1 bunch [80g]	18	0.3	2.4	0.8
Yam					
boiled	100g	133	33.0	1.7	0.3
boiled	1, medium [130g]	173	42.9	2.2	0.4
raw	100g	114	28.2	1.5	0.3

Nuts and Seeds

Specific	Amount	Kcals	Carb	Prot	Fat
Almonds	100g	612	6.9	21.1	55.8
	6 whole [10g]	61	0.7	2.1	5.6
Brazil nuts	100g	682	3.1	14.1	68.2
	6 whole [20g]	136	0.6	2.8	13.6
Cashew nuts					
roasted, salted	100g	611	18.8	20.5	50.9
roasted, salted	10 whole [10g]	61	1.9	2.1	5.1
roasted, salted	25g packet	153	4.7	5.1	12.7
Chestnuts	100g	170	36.6	2.0	2.7
	5 whole [50g]	85	18.3	1.0	1.4
Coconut					
creamed, block	100g	669	7.0	6.0	68.8
dessicated	100g	604	6.4	5.6	62.0
Hazelnuts	100g	650	6.0	14.1	63.5
	10 whole [10g]	65	0.6	1.4	6.4
Macadamia nuts					
salted	100g	748	4.8	7.9	77.6
salted	6 nuts [10g]	75	0.5	0.8	7.8
Mixed nuts	100g	607	7.9	22.9	54.1
	40g packet	243	3.2	9.2	21.6
	50g packet	304	4.0	11.5	27.1
Peanuts					
plain	100g	564	12.5	25.6	46.1
plain	10 whole [10g]	56	1.3	2.6	4.6
roasted, salted	100g	602	7.1	24.5	53.0
roasted, salted	10 whole [10g]	60	0.7	2.5	5.3
roasted, salted	25g packet	151	1.8	6.1	13.3
roasted, salted	40g packet	241	2.8	9.8	21
roasted, salted	50g packet	301	3.6	12.3	26.5

Specific	Amount	Kcals	Carb	Prot	Fat
dry roasted	100g	589	10.3	25.5	49.8
dry roasted	40g packet	236	4.1	10.2	19.9
Pecan nuts	100g	689	5.8	9.2	70.1
	3 nuts [18g]	124	1.0	1.7	12.6
Pine nuts	100g	688	4.0	14.0	68.6
Pistachio nuts	100g	331	4.6	9.9	30.5
	10 nuts [8g]	26	0.4	0.8	2.4
Walnuts	100g	688	3.3	14.7	68.5
	6 halves [20g]	138	0.7	2.9	13.7
Nut-based products					
Marzipan, home-made	100g	461	50.2	10.4	25.8
Marzipan, retail	100g	404	67.6	5.3	14.4
Peanut butter, smooth	100g	623	13.1	22.6	53.7
Peanut butter, smooth	generous spreading [20g]	125	2.6	4.5	10.7
Peanut butter, smooth	thin spreading for bread [12g]	75	1.6	2.7	6.4
Seeds					
Sesame seeds	**100g**	**578**	**0.9**	**18.2**	**58.0**
	1 tbsp [10g]	58	0.1	1.8	5.8
Sunflower seeds	100g	581	18.6	19.8	47.5
	1 tbsp [14g]	81	2.6	2.8	6.7
Seed-based products					
Tahini [sesame seed spread]	100g	607	0.9	18.5	58.9
Tahini [sesame seed spread]	1 heaped tsp [19g]	115	0.2	3.5	11.2

Cereals and Cereal-based Products

Specific	Amount	Kcals	Carb	Prot	Fat
Biscuits					
Cheddars, mini	100g	534	52.9	11.3	30.2
Cheeselets	100g	464	56.9	10.3	21.7
Cheeselets	1 biscuit	5	0.6	0.1	3.3
Chocolate, assorted	100g	524	67.4	5.7	27.6
Club, mint	100g	521	58.9	3.8	30.0
Club, mint	1 biscuit	133	15.1	1.0	7.7
Club, double choc	100g	539	59.3	5.1	29.8
Club, double choc	1 biscuit	127	14.0	1.2	7.0
Digestive	100g	499	67.0	6.5	22.1
Digestive	1 biscuit	73	9.8	1.0	3.3
Digestive with plain chocolate	100g	511	60.8	7.6	26.1
Digestive with plain chocolate	1 biscuit	85	10.0	1.3	4.4
Flapjacks	100g	484	60.4	4.5	26.6
Garibaldis	100g	409	70.5	4.0	9.4
Garibaldis	1 biscuit	45	7.3	0.4	1.0
Gingernut	100g	456	79.1	5.6	15.2
Hob nobs	100g	490	65.3	7.1	21.9
Hob nobs	1 biscuit	72	9.6	1.0	3.2
Homemade	100g	463	64.3	6.2	21.9
Jaffa cakes	100g	363	67.8	3.5	10.5
Sandwich	100g	513	69.2	5.0	25.9
Semi-sweet	100g	457	74.8	6.7	16.6
Short-sweet	100g	469	62.2	6.2	23.4
Wafer, filled	100g	535	66.0	4.7	29.9
Oatcakes	100g	441	63.0	10.0	18.3
Shortbread	100g	498	63.9	5.9	26.1

Specific	Amount	Kcals	Carb	Prot	Fat
Bran					
Wheat	100g	206	26.8	14.1	5.5
Wheat	1 tbsp [7g]	14	1.9	1.0	0.4
Bread					
Brown, average	100g	218	44.3	8.5	2.0
Brown, average	25g slice	55	1.8	2.0	0.5
Chapatis, made with fat	100g	328	48.3	8.1	12.8
Chapatis, made with fat	1 [60g]	197	29.0	4.9	7.7
Chapatis, made without fat	100g	202	43.7	7.3	1.0
Chapatis, made without fat	1 [55g]	111	24.0	4.0	0.6
Croissants	100g	360	38.3	8.3	20.3
Croissants	1, average, plain [50g]	180	19.2	4.2	10.2
Crumpets, toasted	100g	199	43.4	6.7	1.0
Crumpets, toasted	1 [40g]	80	17.4	2.7	0.4
Currant	100g	289	50.7	7.5	7.6
Currant	30g slice	87	15.2	2.3	2.3
Granary	100g	235	46.3	9.3	2.7
Granary	25g slice	59	11.6	2.3	0.7
Hovis	100g	212	41.5	9.5	2.0
Hovis	25g slice	53	10.4	2.4	0.5
Malt	100g	268	56.8	8.3	2.4
Malt	35g slice	94	19.9	2.9	0.8
Naan	100g	336	50.1	8.9	12.5
Naan	160g portion	538	80.2	14.2	20.0
Pitta	100g	265	57.9	9.2	1.2
Pitta	75g pitta	199	43.4	6.9	0.9
Pitta	95g pitta	252	55.0	8.7	1.1
Rolls, brown, crusty	100g	255	50.4	10.3	2.8
Rolls, brown, crusty	1 roll [48g]	122	22.7	4.9	1.3
Rolls, brown, soft	100g	268	51.8	10.0	2.8
Rolls, brown, soft	1 roll [43g]	115	22.3	4.3	1.2
Rolls, hamburger buns	100g	264	48.8	9.1	5.0
Rolls, hamburger buns	1 roll [50g]	132	24.4	4.6	2.5

Calorie Values

Specific	Amount	Kcals	Carb	Prot	Fat
Rolls, white, crusty	100g	280	57.6	10.9	2.3
Rolls, white, crusty	1 roll [50g]	140	28.8	5.5	1.2
Rolls, white, soft	100g	268	51.6	9.2	4.2
Rolls, white, soft	1 roll [45g]	121	23.2	4.4	1.9
Rolls, wholemeal	100g	241	48.3	9.0	2.9
Rolls, wholemeal	1 roll [45g]	108	21.7	4.1	1.3
Rye	100g	219	45.8	8.3	1.7
Rye	25g slice	55	11.5	2.1	0.4
Vitbe	100g	229	43.4	9.7	3.1
Vitbe	25g slice	57	10.9	2.4	0.8
White, 'with added fibre'	100g	230	49.6	7.6	1.5
White, 'with added fibre'	25g slice	58	12.4	1.9	0.4
White, average	100g	235	49.3	8.4	1.9
White, average	25g slice	59	12.3	2.1	0.5
White, french stick	100g	270	55.4	9.6	2.7
White, french stick	2-inch stick [40g]	108	22.2	3.8	1.1
White, fried	100g	503	48.5	7.9	32.2
White, fried	35g slice	176	17.0	2.8	11.3
White, sliced	100g	217	46.8	7.6	1.3
White, sliced	25g slice	54	11.7	1.9	0.3
Wholemeal, average	100g	215	41.6	9.2	2.5
Wholemeal, average	25g slice	54	10.4	2.3	0.6
Breakfast cereal					
All-Bran	100g	261	46.6	14.0	3.4
All-Bran	medium portion [50g]	131	23.3	7.0	1.7
Bran Flakes	100g	318	69.3	10.2	1.9
Bran Flakes	medium portion [40g]	127	27.7	4.1	0.8
Coco Pops	100g	384	74.0	5.3	1.0
Coco Pops	medium portion [30g]	115	22.2	1.6	0.3
Common Sense Oat Bran Flakes	100g	357	85.9	11.0	4.0

Specific	Amount	Kcals	Carb	Prot	Fat
Common Sense Oat Bran Flakes	medium portion [40g]	143	34.4	4.4	1.6
Corn Flakes	100g	360	88.6	7.9	0.7
Corn Flakes	medium portion [40g]	144	35.4	3.2	0.3
Crunchy Nut Corn Flakes	100g	398	93.7	7.4	4.0
Crunchy Nut Corn Flakes	medium portion [40g]	159	37.5	3.0	1.6
Frosties	100g	377	93.7	5.3	0.5
Frosties	medium portion [40g]	151	37.5	2.1	0.2
Fruit 'n Fibre	100g	349	72.1	9.0	4.7
Fruit 'n Fibre	medium portion [40g]	140	28.8	3.6	1.9
Muesli	medium portion [80g]	290	57.8	7.8	4.7
Muesli with no added sugar	100g	366	67.1	10.5	7.8
Muesli with no added sugar	medium portion [80g]	293	53.7	8.4	6.2
Muesli, Swiss style	100g	363	72.2	9.8	5.9
Oat and Wheat Bran	100g	325	67.7	10.6	3.5
Oat and Wheat Bran	medium portion [40g]	130	27.1	4.2	1.4
Porridge, made with milk	medium portion [200g]	232	27.4	9.6	10.2
Porridge, made with water	medium portion [200g]	98	18.0	3.0	2.2
Porridge, with milk	100g	116	13.7	4.8	5.1
Porridge, with water	100g	49	9.0	1.5	1.1
Puffed Wheat	100g	321	67.3	14.2	1.3
Puffed Wheat	medium portion [40g]	128	26.9	5.7	0.5
Raisin Wheats	100g	337	75.4	9.0	2.0

Calorie Values

Specific	Amount	Kcals	Carb	Prot	Fat
Raisin Wheats	medium portion [40g]	135	30.2	3.6	0.8
Ready Brek	100g	373	68.6	11.4	7.8
Ready Brek	medium portion [180g]	671	123.5	20.5	14.0
Rice Krispies	100g	369	89.7	6.1	0.9
Rice Krispies	medium portion [30g]	111	26.9	1.8	0.3
Ricicles	100g	381	95.7	4.3	0.5
Ricicles	medium portion [30g]	114	28.7	1.3	0.2
Shredded Wheat	100g	325	68.3	10.6	3.0
Shredded Wheat	1 piece [22g]	72	304	15.0	2.3
Shreddies	100g	331	74.1	10.1	1.5
Shreddies	medium portion [50g]	166	37.1	5.1	0.8
Smacks	100g	386	89.6	8.0	2.0
Smacks	medium portion [40g]	154	35.8	3.2	0.8
Special K	100g	377	81.7	15.3	1.0
Special K	medium portion [30g]	113	24.5	4.6	0.3
Start	100g	355	81.7	7.9	1.7
Start	medium portion [40g]	142	32.7	3.2	0.7
Sugar Puffs	100g	348	84.5	5.9	0.8
Sugar Puffs	medium portion [40g]	139	33.8	2.4	0.3
Sultana Bran	100g	303	67.8	8.5	1.6
Sultana Bran	medium portion [50g]	121	33.9	4.3	0.8
Weetabix	100g	352	75.7	11.0	2.7
Weetabix	1 piece [20g]	70	15.1	2.2	0.5
Weetaflakes	100g	359	79.3	9.2	2.8

Specific	Amount	Kcals	Carb	Prot	Fat
Weetaflakes	medium portion [40g]	144	31.7	3.7	1.1
Weetos	100g	372	86.1	6.1	2.7
Weetos	medium portion [40g]	149	34.4	2.4	1.1
Buns					
Chelsea	100g	366	56.1	7.8	13.8
Chelsea	1 bun [78g]	285	43.8	6.1	10.8
Currant	100g	296	52.7	7.6	7.5
Currant	1 bun [60g]	178	31.6	4.6	4.5
Hot cross	100g	310	58.5	7.4	6.8
Hot cross	1 bun [50g]	155	29.3	3.7	3.4
Cakes					
Battenburg	100g	370	50.0	5.9	17.5
Battenburg	40g slice	148	20	2.4	7.0
Chocolate Krispie, individual	100g	464	73.1	5.6	18.6
Chocolate Krispie, individual	1 cake [25g]	116	18.3	1.4	4.7
Doughnuts, jam	100g	336	48.8	5.7	14.5
Doughnuts, jam	1 [75g]	252	3.4	4.3	10.9
Doughnuts, ring	100g	397	47.2	6.1	21.7
Doughnuts, ring	1 [60g]	238	28.3	3.7	13.0
Eclairs	100g	396	26.1	5.6	30.6
Eclairs	1 [90g]	356	23.5	5.0	27.5
Fancy Iced, individual	100g	407	68.8	3.8	14.9
Fancy Iced, individual	1 cake [30g]	122	20.6	1.1	4.5
Fruit, plain	100g	354	57.9	5.1	12.9
Fruit, plain	90g slice	319	52.1	4.6	11.6
Fruit, rich	100g	341	59.6	3.8	11.0
Fruit, rich	70g slice	239	41.7	2.7	7.7
Fruit, rich, iced	100g	356	62.7	4.1	11.4
Fruit, rich, iced	70g slice	249	43.9	2.9	8.0
Fruit, wholemeal	100g	363	52.8	6.0	15.7

Calorie Values

Specific	Amount	Kcals	Carb	Prot	Fat
Fruit, wholemeal	90g slice	327	47.5	5.4	14.1
Gateau	100g	337	43.4	5.7	16.8
Gateau	85g slice	286	36.9	4.8	14.3
Madeira	100g	393	58.4	5.4	16.9
Madeira	40g slice	157	23.4	2.2	6.8
Sponge, basic	100g	459	52.4	6.4	26.3
Sponge, basic	53g slice	243	22.5	2.8	11.3
Sponge, fatless	100g	294	53.0	10.1	6.1
Sponge, fatless	53g slice	156	28.1	5.4	3.2
Sponge, jam filled	100g	302	64.2	4.2	4.9
Sponge, jam, filled	65g slice	196	41.7	2.7	3.2
Sponge, butter icing	100g	490	52.4	4.5	30.6
Sponge, butter icing	65g slice	319	34.1	2.9	19.9
Swiss Rolls, chocolate, individual	100g	337	58.1	4.3	11.3
Swiss Rolls, chocolate, individual	1 roll [26g]	88	16.3	1.2	2.9
Teacakes	100g	329	58.3	8.9	8.3
Teacakes	1 [60g]	197	35.0	5.3	5.0
Crackers					
Cream	100g	440	68.3	9.5	16.3
Cream	1 [7g]	31	4.8	0.7	1.1
Wholemeal	100g	413	72.1	10.1	11.3
Wholemeal	1 [15g]	62	10.8	1.5	1.7
Crispbread					
Rye	100g	321	70.6	9.4	2.1
Rye	1 [10g]	32	7.1	0.9	0.2
Custard powder	100g	354	92.0	0.6	0.7
Flour					
Chapati brown	100g	333	73.7	11.5	1.2
Chapati, brown	1 level tbsp [20g]	67	14.7	2.3	0.2
Chapati white	100g	335	77.6	9.8	0.5
Chapati, white	1 level tbsp [20g]	67	15.5	2.0	0.1
Cornflour	100g	354	92.0	0.6	0.7

Specific	Amount	Kcals	Carb	Prot	Fat
Cornflour	1 level tbsp [20g]	71	18	0.1	0.1
Rye flour	100g	335	75.9	8.2	2.0
Rye flour	1 level tbsp [20g]	67	15.2	1.6	0.4
Soya, full fat	100g	447	23.5	36.8	23.5
Soya, full fat	1 level tbsp [20g]	89	4.7	7.4	4.7
Soya, low-fat	100g	352	28.2	45.3	7.2
Soya, low-fat	1 level tbsp [20g]	70	5.6	9.1	1.4
Wheat , brown	100g	323	68.5	12.6	1.8
Wheat, brown	1 level tbsp [20g]	65	13.7	2.5	0.4
Wheat, white, breadmaking	100g	341	75.3	11.5	1.4
Wheat, white, breadmaking	1 level tbsp [20g]	68	15.1	2.3	0.5
Wheat, white, plain	100g	341	77.7	9.4	1.3
Wheat, white, plain	1 level tbsp [20g]	68	15.5	1.9	0.3
Wheat, white, self-raising	100g	330	75.6	8.9	1.2
Wheat, white, self-raising	1 level tbsp [20g]	66	15.1	1.8	0.2
Wheat, wholemeal	100g	310	63.9	12.7	2.2
Wheat, wholemeal	1 level tbsp [20g]	62	12.8	2.5	0.4
Noodles					
Egg, raw	100g	391	71.7	12.1	8.2
Egg, boiled	100g	62	13.0	2.2	0.5
Egg, boiled	300g packet	186	39	6.6	1.5
Oatmeal					
raw	100g	375	66.0	11.2	9.2
Pancakes					
Scotch	100g	292	43.6	5.8	11.7
Scotch	1, [50g]	146	21.8	2.9	5.9
Pasta					
Macaroni, raw	100g	348	75.8	12.0	1.8
Macaroni, boiled	100g	86	18.5	3.0	0.5
Macaroni, boiled	medium portion [230g]	198	42.6	6.9	1.2
Spaghetti, white, raw	100g	342	74.1	12.0	1.8

Calorie Values

Specific	Amount	Kcals	Carb	Prot	Fat
Spaghetti, white, boiled	100g	104	22.2	3.6	0.7
Spaghetti, boiled	medium portion [230g]	239	51.1	8.3	1.6
Spaghetti, wholemeal, raw	100g	324	66.2	13.4	2.5
Spaghetti, wholemeal, boiled	100g	113	23.2	4.7	0.9
Spaghetti, wholemeal, boiled	medium portion [230g]	260	53.4	10.8	2.1
Pastries					
Cream Horns	100g	435	25.8	3.8	35.8
Cream Horns	1 [60g]	261	15.5	2.3	21.5
Custard tarts, individual	100g	277	32.4	6.3	14.5
Custard tarts, individual	1 [94g]	260	30.5	5.9	13.6
Danish	100g	374	51.3	5.8	17.6
Danish	1, medium [110g]	411	56.4	6.4	19.4
Eccles cakes	100g	475	59.3	3.9	26.4
Eccles cakes	1 [45g]	214	26.7	1.8	11.9
Greek	100g	322	40.0	4.7	17.0
Jam tarts	100g	380	62.0	3.3	13.0
Jam tarts	90g slice	342	55.8	3.0	11.7
Mince pies, individual	100g	423	59.0	4.3	20.4
Mince pies, individual	1 [48g]	203	28.3	1.2	9.8
Flaky, raw	100g	424	34.8	4.2	30.7
Flaky, cooked	100g	560	45.9	5.6	40.6
Shortcrust, raw	100g	449	46.8	5.7	27.9
Shortcrust, cooked	100g	521	54.2	6.6	32.3
Wholemeal, raw	100g	431	38.5	7.7	28.4
Wholemeal, cooked	100g	499	44.6	8.9	32.9
Puddings					
Blackcurrant pie, pastry top and bottom	100g	262	34.5	3.1	13.3
Blackcurrant pie, pastry top and bottom	120g portion	314	41.4	3.7	16.0

Specific	Amount	Kcals	Carb	Prot	Fat
Bread pudding	100g	297	49.7	5.9	9.6
Bread pudding	170g portion	505	84.5	10.0	16.3
Christmas pudding, home made	100g [average portion]	291	49.5	4.6	9.7
Christmas pudding, retail	100g [average portion]	329	56.3	3.0	11.8
Crumble, fruit	100g	198	34.0	2.0	6.9
Crumble, fruit	170g portion	337	57.8	3.4	11.7
Crumble, fruit, wholemeal	100g	193	31.7	2.6	7.1
Crumble, fruit, wholemeal	170g portion	328	53.9	4.4	12.1
Fruit pie, top crust only	100g	186	28.7	2.0	7.9
Fruit pie, top crust only	120g portion	223	34.4	2.4	9.4
Fruit pie, pastry top and bottom	100g	260	34.0	3.0	13.3
Fruit pie, pastry top and bottom	120g portion	312	40.8	3.6	16.0
Fruit pie, individual	100g	369	56.7	4.3	15.5
Fruit pie, individual	1 [50g]	185	28.4	2.2	7.8
Fruit pie, wholemeal, top crust only	100g	183	26.6	2.6	8.1
Fruit pie, wholemeal, top crust only	120g portion	220	31.9	3.1	9.7
Fruit pie, wholemeal, pastry top and bottom	100g	251	30.0	4.0	13.6
Fruit pie, wholemeal, pastry top and bottom	120g slice	301	36	4.8	16.3
Lemon meringue pie	100g	319	45.9	4.5	14.4
Lemon meringue pie	120g slice	383	55.1	5.4	17.3
Pancakes, sweet, made with whole milk	100g	301	35.0	5.9	16.2
Pancakes, sweet, made with whole milk	110g portion	331	38.5	6.5	17.8
Pie, with pie filling	100g	273	34.6	3.2	14.5
Pie, with pie filling	120g portion	328	41.5	3.8	17.4

Calorie Values

Specific	Amount	Kcals	Carb	Prot	Fat
Sponge pudding	100g	340	45.3	5.8	16.3
Sponge pudding	170g portion	578	77	9.8	27.7
Treacle tart	100g	368	60.4	3.7	14.1
Treacle tart	120g portion	322	72.5	4.4	16.9
Rice					
Brown, raw	100g	357	81.3	6.7	2.8
Brown, boiled	100g	141	32.1	2.6	1.1
Brown, boiled	medium portion [150g]	212	48.2	3.9	1.7
Savoury, raw	100g	415	77.4	8.4	10.3
Savoury, cooked	100g	142	26.3	2.9	3.5
Savoury, cooked	medium portion [150g]	213	39.5	4.4	5.3
White, easy cook, raw	100g	383	85.8	7.3	3.6
White, easy cook, boiled	100g	138	30.9	2.6	1.3
White, easy cook, boiled	medium portion [150g]	207	46.4	3.9	2.0
White, fried in lard	100g	131	25.0	2.2	3.2
White, fried in lard	300g portion	393	75.0	6.6	9.6
Sago					
raw	100g	355	94.0	0.2	0.2
Cauliflower cheese	100g	105	5.1	5.9	6.9
main dish	200g portion	210	10.2	11.8	13.8
side dish	90g portion	95	4.6	5.3	6.2
Savouries					
Dumplings	100g	208	24.5	2.8	11.7
Macaroni cheese	100g	178	13.6	7.3	10.8
Macaroni cheese	300g portion	534	40.8	21.9	32.4
Pancakes, savoury, made with whole milk	100g	273	24.0	6.3	17.5
Ravioli, in tomato sauce	100g	70	10.3	3.0	2.2
Ravioli, in tomato sauce	200g portion	140	20.6	6.0	4.4
Risotto, plain	100g	224	34.4	3.0	9.3
Risotto, plain	300g portion	672	103.2	9.0	27.9

Specific	Amount	Kcals	Carb	Prot	Fat
Samosas, meat	100g	593	17.9	5.1	56.1
Samosas, vegetable	100g	472	22.3	3.1	41.8
Spaghetti, canned in tomato sauce	100g	64	14.1	1.9	0.4
Spaghetti, canned in tomato sauce	125g portion	80	17.6	2.4	0.5
Stuffing, sage and onion	100g	231	20.4	5.2	14.8
Stuffing mix	100g	338	67.2	9.9	5.2
Stuffing mix, made with water	100g	97	19.3	2.8	1.5
Yorkshire pudding	100g	208	24.7	6.6	9.9
Scones					
Fruit	100g	316	52.9	7.3	9.8
Plain	100g	362	53.8	7.2	14.6
Wholemeal	100g	326	43.1	5.8	11.7
Tapioca					
raw	100g	359	95.0	0.4	0.1
Wheatgerm	100g	357	44.7	26.7	9.2

Eggs and Egg-based Products

Specific	Amount	Kcals	Carb	Prot	Fat
Chicken's egg					
boiled	100g	147	trace	12.5	10.8
boiled	1, size 1 [67g]	98	trace	8.4	7.2
boiled	1, size 2 [61g]	90	trace	7.6	6.6
boiled	1, size 3 [57g]	84	trace	7.1	6.2
boiled	1, size 4 [47g]	69	trace	5.9	5.1
fried in vegetable oil	100g	179	trace	13.6	13.9
fried in vegetable oil	1, average [60g]	107	trace	8.2	8.3
poached	100g	147	trace	12.5	10.8
poached	1, average [50g]	74	trace	6.3	5.4
scrambled, with milk	100g	247	0.6	10.7	22.6
scrambled, with milk	2 eggs [120g]	296	0.7	12.8	27.1
white, raw	100g	36	trace	9.0	trace
whole, raw	100g	147	trace	12.5	10.8
whole, raw	1, size 1 [67g]	98	trace	8.4	7.2
whole, raw	1, size 2 [61g]	90	trace	7.6	6.6
whole, raw	1, size 3 [57g]	84	trace	7.1	6.2
whole, raw	1, size 4 [47g]	69	trace	5.9	5.1
yolk, raw	100g	339	trace	16.1	30.5
Duck egg					
whole, raw	100g	163	trace	14.3	11.8
whole, raw	1, average [75g]	122	trace	17.2	14.2
Egg-based dessert					
Meringue, with cream	100g	376	40.0	3.3	23.6
Meringue, with cream	1 [28g]	105	11.2	0.9	6.6
Meringue, without cream	100g	379	95.4	5.3	trace
Meringue, without cream	1 [8g]	30	7.6	0.4	trace
Egg-based dish					
Egg fried rice	100g	208	25.7	4.2	10.6

Specific	Amount	Kcals	Carb	Prot	Fat
Egg-fried rice	300g portion	624	77.1	12.6	31.8
Omelette, cheese	100g	266	trace	15.9	22.6
Omelette, cheese	2-egg [180g]	479	trace	28.6	40.7
Omelette, plain	100g	191	trace	10.9	16.4
Omelette, plain	2-egg [120g]	229	trace	13.1	19.7
Quiche, cheese and egg	100g	314	17.3	12.5	22.2
Quiche, cheese and egg	70g slice	220	12.1	8.8	15.5
Quiche, cheese and egg	120g slice	377	20.8	15.0	26.6
Quiche, cheese and egg	190g slice	597	32.9	23.8	42.2
Quiche, cheese and egg, wholemeal	100g	308	14.5	13.2	22.4
Quiche, cheese and egg, wholemeal	70g slice	216	10.2	9.2	15.7
Quiche, cheese and egg, wholemeal	120g slice	370	17.4	15.8	26.9
Quiche, cheese and egg, wholemeal	190g slice	585	27.6	25.1	42.6
Scotch egg	100g	251	13.1	12.0	17.1
Scotch egg	1, average [120g]	301	15.7	14.4	20.5

Milk and Dairy Products

Specific	Amount	Kcals	Carb	Prot	Fat
Butter	100g	737	trace	0.5	81.7
thin spreading	[7g]	52	trace	trace	2.9
thick spreading	[12g]	88	trace	0.1	9.8
restaurant portion	[20g]	147	trace	0.1	16.3
Cheese					
Brie	100g	319	trace	19.3	26.9
Brie	40g portion	128	trace	7.7	10.8
Camembert	100g	297	trace	20.9	23.7
Camembert	40g portion	119	trace	8.4	9.5
Cheddar, average	100g	412	0.1	25.5	34.4
Cheddar, average	20g portion	82	trace	5.1	6.9
Cheddar, average	40g portion	165	trace	10.2	13.8
Cheddar, average	60g portion	247	0.1	15.3	20.6
Cheddar, vegetarian	100g	425	trace	25.8	35.7
Cheddar, vegetarian	40g portion	170	trace	10.3	14.3
Cheddar-type, reduced fat	100g	261	trace	31.5	15.0
Cheddar-type, reduced fat	40g portion	104	trace	12.6	6.0
Cheese spread	100g	276	4.4	13.5	22.8
Cheese spread	40g portion	110	1.8	5.4	9.1
Cottage cheese, plain	100g	98	2.1	13.8	3.9
Cottage cheese, plain	112g pot	110	2.4	2.0	4.4
Cottage cheese, reduced fat	100g	78	3.3	13.3	1.4
Cottage cheese, reduced fat	112g pot	87	3.7	1.5	1.6
Cottage cheese, with additions	100g	95	2.6	12.8	3.8
Cottage cheese, with additions	112g pot	106	2.9	14.3	4.3

168

Specific	Amount	Kcals	Carb	Prot	Fat
Cream cheese	100g	439	trace	3.1	47.4
Cream cheese	30g portion	132	trace	0.9	14.2
Danish Blue	100g	347	trace	20.1	29.6
Danish Blue	40g portion	139	trace	8.0	11.8
Edam	100g	333	trace	26.0	25.4
Edam	40g portion	133	trace	10.4	10.2
Feta	100g	250	1.5	15.6	20.2
Feta	20g portion	50	0.3	3.1	4.0
Fromage Frais, fruit	100g	131	13.8	6.8	5.8
Fromage Frais, fruit	60g pot	79	8.3	4.1	3.5
Fromage Frais, plain	100g	113	5.7	6.8	7.1
Fromage Frais, plain	60g pot	68	3.4	4.1	4.3
Fromage Frais, low-fat	100g	58	6.8	7.7	0.2
Fromage Frais, low-fat	60g pot	35	4.1	4.6	0.1
Gouda	100g	375	trace	24.0	31.0
Gouda	40g portion	150	trace	9.6	12.4
Hard cheese, average	100g	405	0.1	24.7	34.0
Hard cheese, average	40g portion	162	trace	9.9	13.6
Parmesan	100g	452	trace	39.4	32.7
Parmesan	10g portion	45	trace	3.9	3.3
Processed, plain	100g	330	0.9	20.8	27.0
Processed, plain	20g slice	66	0.2	4.2	5.4
Soft cheese, full fat	100g	313	trace	8.6	31.0
Soft cheese, full fat	55g portion	172	trace	4.7	17.1
Soft cheese, medium fat	100g	179	3.1	9.2	14.5
Stilton	100g	411	0.1	22.7	35.5
Stilton	40g portion	164	trace	9.1	14.2
White, average	100g	376	0.1	23.4	31.3
White, average	40g portion	150	trace	9.4	12.5
Cream, fresh					
clotted	100g	586	2.3	1.6	63.5
clotted	150g carton	879	3.5	2.4	95.3
double	100g	449	2.7	1.7	48.0
double	150g small	674	4.1	2.6	72.0

Calorie Values

Specific	Amount	Kcals	Carb	Prot	Fat
half	100g	148	4.3	3.0	13.3
half	150g carton	222	6.5	4.5	20.0
single	100g	198	4.1	2.6	19.1
single	150g carton	297	6.2	3.9	28.7
soured	100g	205	3.8	2.9	19.9
soured	150g carton	308	5.7	4.4	30.0
whipping	100g	373	3.1	2.0	39.3
whipping	150g carton	560	4.7	3.0	59.0
Cream, imitation					
Dessert Top	100g	291	6.0	2.4	28.8
Dessert Top	15g portion	44	0.9	0.4	4.3
Dream Topping, made with semi-skimmed milk	100g	166	12.2	3.9	11.7
Dream Topping, made with semi-skimmed milk	15g portion	25	1.8	0.6	1.8
Dream Topping, made with whole milk	100g	182	12.1	3.8	13.5
Dream Topping, made with whole milk	15g portion	27	1.8	0.6	2.0
Elmlea, double	15g portion	68	0.5	0.4	7.2
Elmlea, double	100g	454	3.2	2.5	48.0
Elmlea, single	100g	190	4.1	3.2	18.0
Elmlea, single	15g portion	28.5	0.6	0.5	2.7
Elmlea, whipping	100g	319	3.2	2.5	33.0
Elmlea, whipping	15g portion	48	0.5	0.4	5.0
Tip Top	100g	110	8.5	5.0	6.5
Tip Top	15g portion	17	1.3	0.8	1.0
Cream, sterilised					
canned	100g	239	3.7	2.5	23.9
canned	15g portion	36	0.6	0.4	3.6
Cream, UHT					
canned spray	100g	309	3.5	1.9	32.0
canned spray	15g portion	46.4	0.5	0.3	4.8
Dairy/Fat spread	100g	662	trace	0.4	73.4

Specific	Amount	Kcals	Carb	Prot	Fat
average portion	10g spreading	66	trace	trace	7.3
Dessert					
Cheesecake	100g	242	33.0	5.7	10.6
Cheesecake	110g slice	266	36.3	6.3	11.7
Custard, made with skimmed milk	100g	79	16.8	3.8	0.1
Custard, made with skimmed milk	150g portion	119	25.2	5.7	0.2
Custard, made with whole milk	100g	117	16.6	3.7	4.5
Custard, made with whole milk	150g portion	176	25	5.6	6.8
Instant dessert, made with skimmed milk	100g	97	14.9	3.1	3.2
Instant dessert, made with skimmed milk	120g portion	116	17.9	3.7	3.8
Instant dessert, made with whole milk	100g	125	14.8	3.1	6.3
Instant dessert, made with whole milk	120g portion	150	22.2	4.7	9.5
Milk pudding, made with skimmed milk	100g	93	20.1	4.0	0.2
Milk pudding, made with skimmed milk	200g portion	186	40.2	8.0	0.4
Milk pudding, made with whole milk	100g	129	19.9	3.9	4.3
Milk pudding, made with whole milk	200g portion	258	39.8	7.8	8.6
Mousse, chocolate	100g	139	19.9	4.0	5.4
Mousse, chocolate	60g pot	83	11.9	2.4	3.2
Mousse, fruit	100g	137	18.0	4.5	5.7
Mousse, fruit	60g pot	82.2	10.8	2.7	3.4
Rice pudding, canned	100g	89	14.0	3.4	2.5
Rice pudding, canned	200g portion	178	28.0	6.8	5.0

Calorie Values

Specific	Amount	Kcals	Carb	Prot	Fat
Trifle, home-made	100g	160	22.3	3.6	6.3
Trifle, home-made	170g portion	272	37.9	6.1	10.7
Trifle, home-made, with fresh cream	100g	166	19.5	2.4	9.2
Trifle, home-made, with fresh cream	170g portion	282	33.2	4.1	15.6
Ice cream					
Choc ice	100g	277	28.1	3.5	17.5
Choc ice	50g bar	139	14.1	1.8	8.8
Cornetto	100g	260	34.5	3.7	12.9
Cornetto	75g cone	195	25.9	2.8	9.6
Dairy, flavoured	100g	179	24.7	3.5	8.0
Dairy, flavoured	60g portion	107	14.8	2.1	4.8
Dairy, vanilla	100g	194	24.4	3.6	9.8
Dairy, vanilla	60g portion	116	14.6	2.2	5.9
Lemon sorbet	100g	131	34.2	0.9	trace
Lemon sorbet	60g portion	6.6	20.5	0.5	trace
Non-dairy, flavoured	100g	166	23.2	3.1	7.4
Non-dairy, flavoured	60g portion	100	13.9	1.9	4.4
Non-dairy, vanilla	100g	178	23.1	3.2	8.7
Non-dairy, vanilla	60g portion	107	13.9	1.9	5.1
Ice cream dessert					
Arctic roll	100g	200	33.3	4.1	6.6
Arctic roll	70g slice	140	23.3	2.9	4.6
assorted, average	100g	227	22.8	3.3	14.2
assorted, average	45g portion	102	10.3	1.5	6.4
Chocolate nut sundae	100g	278	34.2	3.0	15.3
Chocolate nut sundae	70g portion	195	23.9	2.1	10.7
Ice cream mix					
prepared	100g	182	25.1	4.1	7.9
Milk, condensed					
skimmed, sweetened	100g	267	60.0	10.0	0.2
whole, sweetened	100g	333	55.5	8.5	10.1
Milk, dried					

Specific	Amount	Kcals	Carb	Prot	Fat
skimmed	100g	348	52.9	36.1	0.6
skimmed, with vegetable fat	100g	487	42.6	23.3	25.9
Milk, evaporated					
whole	100g	151	8.5	8.4	9.4
whole	170g can	257	14.5	14.3	16.0
Milk, flavoured					
mixed flavours, skimmed	100g	68	10.6	3.6	1.5
mixed flavours, skimmed	1/2 pint [293g]	199	31.1	10.6	4.4
Milk, goat's					
pasteurised	100g	60	4.4	3.1	3.5
pasteurised	1 pint [585g]	351	25.7	18.1	20.5
Milk, semi-skimmed					
pasteurised	100g	46	5.0	3.3	1.6
pasteurised	1 pint [585g]	269	29.3	19.3	9.4
pasteurised	30g portion for tea/coffee	14	1.5	1.0	0.5
fortified plus smp	100g	51	5.8	3.7	1.6
fortified plus smp	1 pint [585g]	298	33.9	21.6	9.4
UHT	100g	46	4.8	3.3	1.7
UHT	1 pint [585g]	269	28.1	19.3	9.9
Milk, sheep's					
raw	100g	95	5.1	5.4	6.0
raw	1 pint [585g]	556	29.8	31.6	35.1
pasteurised	100g	33	5.0	3.3	0.1
pasteurised	1 pint [585g]	193	29.3	19.3	0.
Milk, skimmed					
pasteurised	30g serving for tea or coffee	10	1.5	1.0	trace
fortified plus smp	100g	39	6.0	3.8	0.1
fortified plus smp	1 pint [585g]	228	35.1	22.2	0.6
UHT fortified	100g	35	5.0	3.5	0.2
Milk, soya					
plain	100g	32	0.8	2.9	1.9

Calorie Values

Specific	Amount	Kcals	Carb	Prot	Fat
plain	1 pint [585g]	187	4.7	17.0	11.1
flavoured	100g	40	3.6	2.8	1.7
flavoured	1 pint [585g]	236	21.1	16.4	9.0
Milk, whole					
pasteurised	100g	66	4.8	3.2	3.9
pasteurised	1 pint [585g]	386	28.1	18.7	22.8
pasteurised	30g serving for tea or coffee	20	1.4	1.0	1.2
sterilised	100g	66	4.5	3.5	3.9
sterilised	1 pint [585g]	386	26.3	20.5	22.8
UHT, fortified	1 pint [585g]	205	29.3	20.5	1.2
Yoghurt					
drinking	100g	62	13.1	3.1	trace
drinking	210g [200ml] carton	130	27.5	6.5	trace
Greek, cows	100g	115	2.0	6.4	9.1
Greek, cow's	150g carton	173	3.0	9.6	13.7
Greek, sheep's	100g	106	5.6	4.4	7.5
Greek, sheep's	150g carton	159	8.4	6.6	11.3
Low-calorie	100g	41	6.0	4.3	0.2
Low-calorie	150g carton	61.5	9.0	6.5	0.3
Low-fat, flavoured	100g	90	17.9	3.8	0.9
Low-fat, flavoured	150g carton	135	26.9	5.7	1.4
Low-fat, fruit	100g	90	17.9	4.1	0.7
Low-fat, fruit	150g carton	135	26.9	6.2	1.1
Low-fat, plain	100g	56	7.5	5.1	0.8
Low-fat, plain	150g carton	84	11.3	7.7	1.2
Soya	100g	72	3.9	5.0	4.2
Soya	150g carton	108	5.9	7.5	6.3
Whole milk, fruit	150g carton	158	23.6	7.7	4.2
Whole milk, fruit	100g	105	15.7	5.1	2.8
Whole milk, plain	100g	79	7.8	5.7	3.0
Whole milk, plain	150g carton	119	11.7	8.6	4.5

Specific	Amount	Kcals	Carb	Prot	Fat
Yoghurt-based dish					
Tzatziki	100g	66	2.0	3.7	4.9
	50 g portion	33	1.0	1.8	2.4

Fats and Oils

Specific	Amount	Kcals	Carb	Prot	Fat
Animal fat					
Compound cooking fat	100g	894	trace	trace	99.3
Dripping, beef	100g	891	trace	trace	99.0
Lard	100g	891	trace	trace	99.0
Suet, shredded	100g	826	12.1	trace	86.7
Ghee					
Butter	100g	898	trace	trace	99.8
Palm	100g	897	trace	trace	99.7
Vegetable	100g	898	trace	trace	99.8
Oil					
Coconut oil	100g	899	0	trace	99.9
Cod liver oil	100g	899	0	trace	99.9
Corn oil	100g	899	0	trace	99.9
Cottonseed oil	100g	899	0	trace	99.9
Olive oil	100g	899	0	trace	99.9
Palm oil	100g	899	0	trace	99.9
Peanut oil	100g	899	0	trace	99.9
Rapeseed oil	100g	899	0	trace	99.9
Safflower oil	100g	899	0	trace	99.9
Sesame oil	100g	881	0	0.2	99.7
Soya oil	100g	899	0	trace	99.9
Sunflower seed oil	100g	899	0	trace	99.9
Vegetable oil, blended, average	100g	899	0	trace	99.9
Wheatgerm oil	100g	899	0	trace	99.9
Spreading fat					
Butter	100g	737	trace	0.5	81.7
Dairy/fat spread	100g	662	trace	0.4	73.4
Low-fat spread	100g	390	0.5	5.8	40.5

Specific	Amount	Kcals	Carb	Prot	Fat
Margarine, hard, animal and vegetable fat	100g	739	1.0	0.2	81.6
Margarine, hard, vegetable fat only	100g	739	1.0	0.2	81.6
Margarine, soft, animal and vegetable fat	100g	739	1.0	0.2	81.6
Margarine, soft, vegetable fat only	100g	739	1.0	0.2	81.6
Margarine, polyunsaturated	100g	739	1.0	0.2	81.6
Very low-fat spread	100g	273	3.6	8.3	25.0

Savoury Dishes

Specific	Amount	Kcals	Carb	Prot	Fat
Cereal-based dish					
Pizza, cheese and tomato, home-made	100g	235	24.8	9.0	11.8
Pizza, cheese and tomato, home-made	300g portion	705	74.4	27.0	35.4
Cereal/Vegetable dish					
Pancake roll, with vegetable and beansprout filling	100g	217	20.9	6.6	12.5
Pancake roll, with vegetable and beansprout filling	85g roll	184	17.8	5.6	10.6
Egg-based dish					
Omelette, cheese	100g	266	trace	15.9	22.6
Omelette, cheese	2 eggs [180g]	479	trace	28.6	40.7
Omelette, plain	100g	191	trace	10.9	16.4
Omelette, plain	2 eggs [120g]	229	trace	13.1	19.7
Quiche, cheese and egg	100g	314	17.3	12.5	22.2
Quiche, cheese and egg	70g portion	220	12.1	8.8	15.5
Quiche, cheese and egg	120g portion	377	20.8	15.0	26.6
Quiche, cheese and egg	190g portion	597	32.9	23.8	42.2
Quiche, cheese and egg, wholemeal	100g	308	14.5	13.2	22.4
Quiche, cheese and egg, wholemeal	70g portion	216	10.2	9.2	15.7
Quiche, cheese and egg, wholemeal	120g portion	370	17.4	15.8	26.9
Quiche, cheese and egg, wholemeal	190g portion	410	27.6	25.1	42.6
Fish-based dish					
Cod fried in batter	[chip shop] 100g	199	7.5	19.6	10.3

Specific	Amount	Kcals	Carb	Prot	Fat
Cod fried in batter	[chip shop] 190g	378	14.3	37.2	19.6
Cod fried in batter with chips [chip shop]	190g cod, 200g chips	856	75.3	43.6	44.4
Fish cakes, fried	100g	188	15.1	9.1	10.5
Fish cakes, fried	1 fish cake [50g]	94	7.6	4.6	5.3
Fish fingers, fried	100g	233	17.2	13.5	12.7
Fish fingers, fried	1 fish finger [28g]	65	4.8	3.8	3.6
Fish fingers, fried	1 fish finger, jumbo size [60g]	140	10.3	2.3	1.0
Fish fingers, fried, with home-made chips	3 x 28g fingers, 180g chips	535	68.6	18.4	22.9
Fish fingers, fried, with oven chips	3 x 28g fingers, 180g chips	486	68	17.2	18.4
Fish fingers, grilled	100g	214	19.3	15.1	9.0
Fish fingers, grilled	1 finger, [28g]	60	5.4	4.3	2.5
Fish fingers, grilled	1 finger, jumbo size [60g]	128	11.6	9.1	5.4
Fish fingers, grilled, with oven chips	3x28g fingers, 180g chips	471	69.8	18.7	15.1
Fish pie, home-made	100g	105	12.3	8.0	3.0
Fish pie, home-made	250g portion	263	30.8	20.0	7.5
Haddock fried in breadcrumbs	100g	174	3.6	21.4	8.3
Haddock fried in breadcrumbs	120g portion	209	4.3	25.7	10.0
Haddock fried in breadcrumbs with oven chips	120g haddock, 180g chips,	500	57.9	31.5	17.6
Plaice fried in batter [chip shop]	100g	279	14.4	15.8	18.0
Plaice fried in batter [chip shop]	190g portion	530	27.4	30.0	34.2
Plaice fried in batter with chips	190g plaice, 200g chips	1008	88.4	36.4	59.0

Calorie Values

Specific	Amount	Kcals	Carb	Prot	Fat
Scampi, fried in breadcrumbs	100g	316	28.9	12.2	17.6
Scampi, fried in breadcrumbs	150g portion	474	43.4	18.3	26.4
Scampi, fried in breadcrumbs with home-made chips	150g scampi, 180g chips	814	97.6	25.3	38.5
Fish/Rice dish					
Kedgeree, home-made	100g	166	10.5	14.2	7.9
Kedgeree, home-made	300g portion	498	31.5	42.6	23.7
Meat-based dish					
Beef chow mein	100g	136	14.7	6.7	6.0
Beef chow mein	330g portion	449	48.5	22.1	19.8
Beef curry	100g	137	6.3	13.5	6.6
Beef curry	330g portion	452	20.8	44.6	21.8
Beef curry with rice	100g	137	16.9	8.8	4.3
Beef curry with rice	400g portion	548	67.6	35.2	17.2
Beef kheema	100g	413	0.3	18.2	37.7
Beef kheema	250g portion	1032	0.8	45.5	94.3
Beef khoftas	100g	353	3.4	23.3	27.6
Beef khoftas	250g portion	883	8.5	58.3	69.0
Beef sausages, fried, with home-made chips	2 60g sausages, 180g chips	661	72.1	22.5	33.6
Beef sausages, grilled, with boiled potatoes	2 60g sausages, 180g potatoes	448	49.2	18.8	21.0
Beef steak pudding	100g	224	18.8	10.8	12.3
Beef steak pudding	230g portion	515	43.2	24.8	28.3
Beef steak pudding	450g portion	1008	84.6	48.6	5.9
Beef stew	100g	120	4.6	9.7	7.2
Beef stew	330g portion	396	15.2	32.0	23.8
Beefburger, fried, in burger bun	105g beefburger, 50g bun	410	31.8	26.0	20.7
Beefburger, fried, in burger bun with fries	105g burger, 50g bun, 93g fries	670	63.4	29.1	35.1

Specific	Amount	Kcals	Carb	Prot	Fat
Bolognese sauce	100g	145	3.7	8.0	11.1
Bolognese sauce	220g portion	319	8.1	17.6	24.4
Chicken curry	100g	205	3.1	10.2	17.0
Chicken curry	330g portion	677	10.2	4.0	56.1
Chicken curry with rice	100g	144	16.9	7.8	5.5
Chicken curry with rice	400g portion	576	67.6	31.2	22.0
Chicken in white sauce	½ can [210g]	391	7.4	20.0	31.5
Chicken in white sauce, canned	100g	186	3.5	9.5	15.0
Chilli con carne	100g	151	8.3	11.0	8.5
Chilli con carne	220g portion	332	18.3	24.2	18.7
Cottage pie, frozen	100g	110	11.4	5.1	4.7
Cottage pie, frozen	450g portion	495	51.3	22.9	21.2
Curried meat	100g	162	9.1	8.5	10.5
Curried meat	330g portion	535	30.0	28.1	34.7
Hot pot, home-made	100g	144	10.1	9.4	4.5
Hot pot, home-made	330g portion	475	33.3	31.0	14.9
Irish stew	100g	123	9.1	5.3	7.6
Irish stew	330g portion	406	30.0	17.5	25.1
Lamb hot pot, frozen	100g	92	7.9	7.9	3.4
Lamb hot pot, frozen	340g portion	320	28.0	28.0	12.0
Lamb kheema	100g	328	2.3	14.6	29.1
Lamb kheema	250g portion	820	5.8	36.5	72.8
Lasagne	100g	102	12.8	5.0	3.8
Lasagne	450g portion	459	57.6	22.5	17.1
Moussaka, frozen	100g	105	9.9	7.0	4.4
Moussaka, frozen	340g portion	355	34.0	24.0	5.4
Moussaka, home-made	100g	184	7.0	9.1	13.6
Moussaka, home-made	330g portion	607	23.1	30.0	44.9
Mutton biriani	100g	276	25.1	7.5	16.9
Mutton biriani	330g portion	911	82.8	24.8	55.8
Mutton curry	100g	374	3.9	14.9	33.4
Mutton curry	330g portion	1234	12.9	49.2	110.2
Shepherd's pie	100g	118	8.2	8.0	6.2

Calorie Values

Specific	Amount	Kcals	Carb	Prot	Fat
Shepherd's pie	300g portion	354	24.6	24.0	18.6
Spaghetti bolognese	220g sauce, 230g pasta	558	59.2	25.9	26.0
Steak and kidney pie, individual	100g	323	25.6	9.1	21.2
Steak and kidney pie, individual	1 pie [200g]	646	51.2	18.2	42.4
Steak and kidney pie, pastry top only	100g	286	15.9	15.2	18.4
Steak and kidney pie, pastry top only	120g portion	343	19.1	18.2	22.1
Pasta dish					
Macaroni cheese with ham	100g	146	13.3	9.9	5.7
Macaroni cheese with ham	284g serving	460	42.0	31.0	18.0
Macaroni cheese, home-made	100g	178	13.6	7.3	10.8
Macaroni cheese, home-made	300g portion	534	40.8	21.9	32.4
Rice-based dish					
Egg-fried rice	100g	208	25.7	4.2	10.6
Egg-fried rice	300g portion	624	77.1	12.6	31.8
Risotto, plain	100g	224	34.4	3.0	9.3
Risotto, plain	300g portion	672	103.2	9.0	27.9
Vegetable dish					
Cauliflower cheese	100g	105	5.1	5.9	6.9
Cauliflower cheese	side dish [90g]	95	4.6	5.3	6.2
Cauliflower cheese	main course [200g]	210	10.2	11.8	13.8
Vegetable-based dish					
Ratatouille, canned	100g	38	3.0	1.0	2.5
Ratatouille, canned	1/2 can [200g]	76	6.0	2.0	5.0
Vegetable chilli, canned	100g	86	9.1	4.3	3.8
Vegetable chilli, canned	1/2 can [200g]	172	18.2	8.6	7.6

Meats and Meat Dishes

Specific	Amount	Kcals	Carb	Prot	Fat
Bacon					
Collar joint, boiled	100g	325	0	20.4	27.0
Collar joint, boiled	55g portion	179	0	11.2	14.9
Collar joint, raw	100g	319	0	14.6	28.9
Gammon joint, boiled	100g	269	0	24.7	18.9
Gammon joint, boiled	55g portion	148	0	13.6	10.4
Gammon joint, raw	100g	236	0	17.6	18.3
Gammon rasher, grilled	100g	228	0	29.5	12.2
Gammon rasher, grilled	55g portion	125	0	16.2	6.7
Rasher [back], grilled	100g	405	0	25.3	33.8
Rasher [back], grilled	1 rasher [25g]	101	0	6.3	8.5
Rasher [back], raw	100g	428	0	14.2	41.2
Rasher [middle], grilled	100g	416	0	24.9	35.1
Rasher [middle], grilled	1 rasher [40g]	166	0	10.0	14.0
Rasher [middle], raw	100g	425	0	14.3	40.9
Rasher [streaky], grilled	100g	422	0	24.5	36.0
Rasher [streaky], grilled	1 rasher [20g]	84	0	4.9	7.2
Rasher [streaky], raw	100g	414	0	14.6	39.5
Beef					
Brisket, boiled	100g	326	0	27.6	23.9
Brisket, boiled	200g portion	652	0	55.2	47.8
Brisket, raw	100g	252	0	16.8	20.5
Forerib, raw	100g	290	0	16.0	25.1
Forerib, roast	100g	349	0	22.4	28.8
Forerib, roast	120g portion	419	0	26.9	34.6
Mince, raw	100g	221	0	18.8	16.2
Mince, stewed	100g	229	0	23.1	15.2
Mince, stewed	200g portion	458	0	46.2	30.4
Rump steak, fried	100g	246	0	28.6	14.6

Calorie Values

Specific	Amount	Kcals	Carb	Prot	Fat
Rump steak, fried	115g steak	283	0	32.9	16.8
Rump steak, fried	180g steak	443	0	51.5	26.3
Rump steak, grilled	100g	218	0	27.3	12.1
Rump steak, grilled	115g steak	251	0	31.4	13.9
Rump steak, grilled	180g steak	392	0	49.1	21.8
Rump steak, raw	100g	197	0	18.9	13.5
Salted	100g	119	0	27.1	0.4
Silverside, salted, boiled	100g	242	0	28.6	14.2
Silverside, salted, boiled	125g portion	303	0	35.8	17.8
Sirloin, raw	100g	272	0	16.6	22.8
Sirloin, roast	100g	284	0	23.6	21.1
Sirloin, roast	120g portion	341	0	28.3	25.3
Stewing steak, raw	100g	176	0	20.2	10.6
Stewing steak, stewed	100g	223	0	30.9	11.0
Stewing steak, stewed	200g portion	446	0	15.5	5.6
Topside, raw	100g	179	0	19.6	11.2
Topside, roast	100g	214	0	26.6	12.0
Topside, roast	120g portion	256.8	0	31.9	14.4
Beef-based dish					
Beef kheema	100g	413	0.3	18.2	37.7
Beef kheema	250g portion	1032	0.8	45.5	94.3
Beef steak pudding	100g	224	18.8	10.8	12.3
Beef steak pudding	230g portion	515	43.2	24.8	28.3
Beef steak pudding	450g portion	1008	84.6	48.6	55.4
Beef stew, home made	100g	120	4.6	9.7	7.2
Beef stew, home-made	330g portion	396	15.2	32.0	23.8
Bolognese sauce	100g	145	3.7	8.0	11.1
Bolognese sauce	220g portion	319	8.1	17.6	24.4
Chilli con carne	100g	151	8.3	11.0	8.5
Chilli con carne	220g portion	332	18.3	24.2	18.7
Chow mein	100g	136	14.7	6.7	6.0
Chow mein	330g portion	449	48.5	22.1	19.8
Curry	100g	137	6.3	13.5	6.6
Curry	330g portion	452	20.8	44.6	21.8

Specific	Amount	Kcals	Carb	Prot	Fat
Curry with rice	100g	137	16.9	8.8	4.3
Curry with rice	400g portion	548	67.6	35.2	17.2
Stewed steak, canned, with gravy	100g	176	1.0	14.8	12.5
Stewed steak, canned, with gravy	½ can [210g]	370	2.1	31.1	26.3
Beefburgers, frozen, raw	100g	265	5.3	15.2	20.5
Beefburgers, frozen, fried	100g	264	7.0	20.4	17.3
Beefburgers, frozen, fried	1 burger [50g]	132	3.5	10.2	8.7
Corned beef, canned	100g	217	0	26.9	12.1
Chicken and chicken-based dishes					
Breaded, fried in oil	100g	242	14.8	18.0	12.7
Breaded, fried in oil	140g portion	339	20.7	25.2	15.2
Dark meat, boiled	100g	204	0	28.6	9.9
Dark meat, boiled	120g portion	245	0	34.3	11.9
Dark meat, raw	100g	126	0	19.1	5.5
Dark meat, roast	100g	155	0	23.1	6.9
Dark meat, roast	120g portion	186	0	27.7	8.3
Leg quarter, roast	100g	92	0	15.4	3.4
Leg quarter, roast	1 quarter [190g]	175	0	29.3	6.5
Light and dark meat, boiled	100g	183	0	29.2	7.3
Light and dark meat, boiled	120g portion	220	0	35.0	8.8
Light and dark meat, raw	100g	121	0	20.5	4.3
Light and dark meat, roast	100g	148	0	24.8	5.4
Light and dark meat, roast	120g portion	178	0	29.8	6.5
Light meat, boiled	100g	163	0	29.7	4.9
Light meat, boiled	120g portion	196	0	35.6	5.9
Light meat, raw	100g	116	0	21.8	3.2
Light meat, roast	100g	142	0	26.5	4.0
Light meat, roast	120g portion	170	0	31.8	4.8

Calorie Values

Specific	Amount	Kcals	Carb	Prot	Fat
Wing quarter, roast	100g	74	0	12.4	2.7
Wing quarter, roast	1 quarter [190g]	141	0	23.6	5.1
Chicken in white sauce, canned	100g	176	3.5	9.5	15.0
Chicken in white sauce, canned	420g can	780	15.0	40.0	63.0
Curry	100g	205	3.1	10.2	17.0
Curry	330g portion	677	68.3	83.2	56.1
Curry with rice	100g	144	16.9	7.8	5.5
Curry with rice	330g portion	475	55.8	25.7	18.2
Duck					
roast	100g	189	0	25.3	9.7
roast	120g portion	227	0	30.4	11.6
Goose					
roast	100g	319	0	29.3	22.4
roast	120g portion	383	0	35.2	26.9
Grouse					
roast	100g	173	0	31.3	5.3
roast	1 grouse [160g]	277	0	50.1	8.5
Ham					
canned	100g	120	0	18.4	5.1
canned	120g portion	144	0	22.1	6.1
Honey roast	100g	108	2.4	18.2	2.9
Honey roast	30g slice	32	0.7	5.4	0.9
Smoked	100g	94	0.8	17.6	2.3
Smoked	30g slice	28	0.2	5.9	0.7
Hare					
Stewed	100g	192	0	29.9	8.0
Stewed	150g portion	288	0	44.9	12.0
Lamb and lamb dishes					
Breast, raw	100g	378	0	16.7	34.6
Breast, roast	100g	410	0	19.1	37.1
breast, roast	120g portion	492	0	22.9	44.5
Chops, Loin, grilled	100g	355	0	23.5	29.0

Specific	Amount	Kcals	Carb	Prot	Fat
Chops, Loin, grilled	1 chop [90g]	320	0	21.2	26.1
Chops, Loin, raw	100g	377	0	14.6	35.4
Cutlets, grilled	100g	370	0	23.0	30.9
Cutlets, grilled	1 cutlet [50g]	185	0	11.5	15.5
Cutlets, raw	100g	386	0	14.7	36.3
Leg, raw	100g	240	0	17.9	18.7
Leg, roast	100g	266	0	26.1	17.9
Leg, roast	120g portion	319	0	31.2	21.5
Scrag and neck, raw	100g	316	0	15.6	28.2
Scrag and neck, stewed	100g	292	0	25.6	21.1
Scrag and neck, stewed	200g portion	598	0	51.2	42.2
Shoulder, raw	100g	314	0	15.6	28.0
Shoulder, roast	100g	316	0	19.9	26.3
Shoulder, roast	120g portion	379	0	23.9	50.0
Irish stew	100g	123	9.1	5.3	7.6
Irish stew	330g portion	406	30.0	17.5	25.1
Lamb kheema	100g	328	2.3	14.6	29.1
Lamb kheema	250g portion	820	5.8	36.5	72.8
Moussaka	100g	184	7.0	9.1	13.6
Moussaka	330g portion	607	23.1	30.0	44.9
Lamb hot pot, frozen	100g	92	7.9	7.9	3.4
Lamb hot pot, frozen	340g portion	320	28.0	28.0	12.0
Moussaka, frozen	100g	105	9.9	7.0	4.4
Moussaka, frozen	340g portion	355	34.0	24.0	5.4
Meat-based dish					
Cottage pie, frozen	100g	110	11.4	5.1	4.7
Cottage pie, frozen	450g portion	495	51.3	23.0	21.2
Hot pot, home made	100g	114	10.1	9.4	4.5
Hot pot, home made	330g portion	376	33.3	31.0	14.9
Lasagne	100g	102	12.8	5.0	3.8
Lasagne	450g portion	459	57.6	22.5	17.1
Meat curry	100g	162	9.1	8.5	10.5
Meat curry	330g portion	535	30.0	28.1	34.7
Shepherd's pie	100g	118	8.2	8.0	6.2

Calorie Values

Specific	Amount	Kcals	Carb	Prot	Fat
Shepherd's pie	300g portion	354	24.6	24.0	18.6
Meat-based products					
Black pudding, fried	100g	305	15.0	12.9	21.9
Black pudding, fried	120g portion [3 slices]	366	18.0	15.5	26.3
Brawn	100g	153	0	12.4	11.5
Chopped ham and pork, canned	100g	275	1.4	14.4	23.6
Cornish pasty	100g	332	31.1	8.0	20.4
Cornish pasty	1 medium pasty [155g]	515	48.2	12.4	31.6
Faggots	100g	268	15.3	11.1	18.5
Faggots	2 faggots [150g]	402	23.0	16.7	27.8
Frankfurters	100g	274	3.0	9.5	25.0
Frankfurters	1 large [47g]	129	1.4	4.5	11.8
Grillsteaks, grilled	100g	305	0.5	22.1	23.9
Grillsteaks, grilled	1 steak [80g]	244	0.4	17.7	19.1
Haggis, boiled	100g	310	19.2	10.7	21.7
Haggis, boiled	220g portion	682	42.2	23.5	47.7
Liver pâté	100g	316	1.0	13.1	28.9
Liver pâté	40g portion	126	0.4	5.2	11.6
Liver pâté, low-fat	100g	191	2.8	18.0	12.0
Liver pâté, low-fat	40g portion	76	1.1	7.2	4.8
Liver sausage	100g	310	4.3	12.9	26.9
Liver sausage	40g portion	124	1.7	5.2	10.8
Luncheon meat, canned	100g	313	5.5	12.6	26.9
Luncheon meat, canned	20g slice	63	3.3	7.6	16.1
Meat paste	100g	173	3.0	15.2	11.2
Meat paste	40g portion	69	1.2	6.1	4.5
Pepperami	100g	560	1.0	20	52
Pepperami	25g stick	140	0.3	5.0	13
Polony	100g	281	14.2	9.4	21.1
Polony	20g slice	56	2.8	1.9	4.2
Pork pie, individual	100g	376	24.9	9.8	27.0

Specific	Amount	Kcals	Carb	Prot	Fat
Pork pie, individual	1 pie [140g]	526	34.9	13.7	37.8
Salami	100g	491	1.9	19.3	45.2
Salami	1 slice [17g]	83	0.3	3.3	7.7
Sausage roll, flaky pastry	100g	477	32.3	7.1	36.4
Sausage roll, flaky pastry	1, medium [60g]	286	19.4	46.3	21.8
Sausage roll, short pastry	100g	459	37.5	8.0	31.9
Sausage roll, short pastry	1, medium [60g]	275	22.5	4.8	19.1
Saveloy	100g	262	10.1	9.9	20.5
Saveloy	1 saveloy [65g]	170	6.6	6.4	1.6
Steak and kidney pie, individual,pastry top and bottom	1 pie [200g]	646	51.2	18.2	42.4
Steak and kidney pie, individual,pastry top and bottom	100g	323	25.6	9.1	21.2
Steak and kidney pie, pastry top only	100g	286	15.9	15.2	18.4
Steak and kidney pie, pastry top only	120g portion	343	19.1	18.2	22.1
White pudding	100g	450	36.3	7.0	31.8
White pudding	120g portion	540	43.6	8.4	38.2
Sausages, beef, fried	100g	269	14.9	12.9	18.0
Sausages, beef, fried	1 thin [35g]	94	5.2	4.5	6.3
Sausages, beef, fried	1 large [60g]	161	8.9	1.1	10.8
Sausages, beef, grilled	100g	265	15.2	13.0	17.3
Sausages, beef, grilled	1 large [60g]	159	9.1	7.8	10.4
Sausages, beef, grilled	1 thin [35g]	93	5.3	4.6	6.1
Sausages, beef, raw	100g	299	11.7	9.6	24.1
Sausages, pork, fried	100g	317	11.0	13.8	24.5
Sausages, pork, fried	1 thin [35g]	111	3.9	4.8	8.6
Sausages, pork, fried	1 large [60g]	190	6.6	8.3	14.7
Sausages, pork, grilled	100g	318	11.5	13.3	24.6
Sausages, pork, grilled	1 thin [35g]	111	4.0	4.7	8.6
Sausages, pork, grilled	1 large [60g]	191	6.9	8.0	14.8

Calorie Values

Specific	Amount	Kcals	Carb	Prot	Fat
Sausages, pork, low-fat, fried	100g	211	9.1	14.9	13.0
Sausages, pork, low-fat, fried	1 thin [35g]	74	3.2	5.2	4.6
Sausages, pork, low-fat, fried	1 large [60g]	127	5.5	8.9	7.8
Sausages, pork, low-fat, grilled	100g	229	10.8	16.2	13.8
Sausages, pork, low-fat, grilled	1 thin [35g]	80	3.8	5.7	4.8
Sausages, pork, low-fat, grilled	1 large [60g]	137	6.5	9.7	8.3
Sausages, pork, low-fat, raw	100g	166	8.1	12.5	9.5
Sausages, pork, raw	100g	367	9.5	10.6	32.1
Mutton-based dish					
Mutton biriani	100g	276	25.1	7.5	16.9
Mutton biriani	330g portion	911	82.8	24.8	55.8
Mutton curry	100g	374	3.9	14.9	33.4
Mutton curry	330g portion	1234	12.9	49.2	110.2
Offal					
Heart, lamb, raw	100g	119	0	17.1	5.6
Heart, ox, raw	100g	108	0	18.9	3.6
Heart, ox, stewed	100g	179	0	31.4	5.9
Heart, sheep, roast	100g	237	0	26.1	14.7
Kidney, lamb, fried	100g	155	0	24.6	6.3
Kidney, lamb, fried	1 whole [90g]	140	0	22.1	5.7
Kidney, lamb, raw	100g	90	0	16.5	2.7
Kidney, ox, raw	100g	86	0	15.7	2.6
Kidney, ox, stewed	100g	172	0	25.6	7.7
Kidney, ox, stewed	112g portion	193	0	28.7	8.6
Kidney, pig, raw	100g	90	0	16.3	2.7
Kidney, pig, stewed	100g	153	0	24.4	6.1
Kidney, pig, stewed	112g portion	171	0	27.3	6.8

Specific	Amount	Kcals	Carb	Prot	Fat
Liver, calf, coated in flour and fried	100g	254	7.3	26.9	13.2
Liver, calf, coated in oil and fried	40g slice	102	2.9	10.8	5.3
Liver, calf, raw	100g	153	1.9	20.1	7.3
Liver, chicken, coated in flour and fried	100g	194	3.4	20.7	10.9
Liver, chicken, coated in flour and fried	70g portion	136	2.4	14.5	7.6
Liver, chicken, raw	100g	135	0.6	19.1	6.3
Liver, lamb, coated in flour and fried	100g	232	3.9	22.9	14.0
Liver, lamb, coated in oil and fried	40g slice	93	1.6	9.2	16.8
Liver, lamb, raw	100g	179	1.6	20.1	10.3
Liver, ox raw	100g	163	2.2	21.1	7.8
Liver, ox, coated in flour and stewed	100g	198	3.6	24.8	9.5
Liver, ox, coated in flour and stewed	70g portion	139	2.5	17.4	6.7
Liver, pig, coated in flour and stewed	100g	189	3.6	25.6	8.1
Liver, pig, coated in flour and stewed	70 g portion	132	2.5	17.9	5.7
Liver, pig, raw	100g	154	2.1	21.3	6.8
Oxtail, stewed	100g	243	0	30.5	13.4
Oxtail, stewed	330g portion	802	0	100.7	44.2
Sweetbread, lamb, coated in egg and breadcrumbs and fried	100g	230	5.6	19.4	14.6
Sweetbread, lamb, coated in egg and breadcrumbs and fried	70g portion	161	3.9	13.6	10.2
Sweetbread, lamb, raw	100g	131	0	15.3	7.8

Calorie Values

Specific	Amount	Kcals	Carb	Prot	Fat
Tongue, lamb, raw	100g	193	0	15.3	14.6
Tongue, ox, boiled	100g	293	0	19.5	23.9
Tongue, ox, pickled, raw	100g	220	0	15.7	17.5
Tongue, sheep, stewed	100g	289	0	18.2	24.0
Tripe, dressed	100g	60	0	9.4	2.5
Tripe, dressed, stewed in milk	100g	100	0	14.8	4.5
Tripe, dressed, stewed in milk	70g portion	70	0	10.4	3.2
Partridge					
roast	100g	212	0	36.7	7.2
roast	1 [260g]	551	0	95.4	18.7
Pheasant					
roast	100g	213	0	32.2	9.3
roast	1 [430g]	916	0	138.5	40.0
Pigeon					
roast	100g	230	0	27.8	13.2
roast	1 [115g]	265	0	32.0	15.2
Pork					
Belly rashers, grilled	100g	398	0	21.1	34.8
Belly rashers, grilled	110g portion	438	0	23.2	38.3
Belly rashers, raw	100g	381	0	15.3	35.5
Chops, loin, grilled	100g	332	0	28.5	24.2
Chops, loin, grilled	120g portion	398	0	34.2	29.0
Chops, loin, raw	100g	329	0	15.9	29.5
Leg, raw	100g	269	0	16.6	22.5
Leg, roast	100g	286	0	26.9	19.8
Leg, roast	120g portion	343	0	32.3	23.8
Trotters and tails, boiled	100g	280	0	19.8	22.3
Rabbit					
raw	100g	124	0	21.9	4.0
stewed	100g	179	0	27.3	7.7
stewed	200g portion	358	0	54.6	15.4

Specific	Amount	Kcals	Carb	Prot	Fat
Tongue					
canned	100g	213	0	16.0	16.5
Turkey and turkey-based products					
Dark meat, raw	100g	114	0	20.3	3.6
Dark meat, roast	100g	148	0	27.8	4.1
Dark meat, roast	120g portion	178	0	33.4	4.9
Light and dark meat, raw	100g	107	0	21.9	2.2
Light and dark meat, roast	100g	140	0	28.8	2.7
Light and dark meat, roast	120g portion	168	0	34.6	3.2
Light meat, raw	100g	103	0	23.2	1.1
Light meat, roast	100g	132	0	29.8	1.4
Light meat, roast	120g portion	158	0	35.8	1.7
Turkey with ham	100g	123	2.2	19.2	4.1
Turkey with ham	30g slice	37	0.7	5.8	1.2
Veal					
Cutlet, coated in egg and breadcrumbs and fried	100g	215	4.4	31.4	8.1
Cutlet, coated in egg and breadcrumbs and fried	1 cutlet [150g]	323	6.6	47.1	12.2
Fillet, raw	100g	109	0	21.1	2.7
Fillet, roast	100g	230	0	31.6	11.5
Fillet, roast	120g portion	276	0	37.9	13.8
Venison					
Haunch, roast	100g	198	0	35.0	6.4
Haunch, roast	120g portion	238	0	42.0	7.7

Fish and Seafood

Specific	Amount	Kcals	Carb	Prot	Fat
Anchovies					
canned in oil, drained	100g	280	0	25.2	19.9
canned in oil, drained	1 anchovy [3g]	8.4	0	0.8	0.6
canned in oil, drained	50g tin	140	0	12.6	10.0
canned in oil, drained	for pizza [10g]	28	0	2.5	2.0
Cockles					
boiled	100g	48	trace	11.3	0.3
boiled	1 cockle [4g]	2	0	0.5	trace
boiled	142g jar	68	0	16.0	0.4
boiled	25g portion	12	0	2.8	0.1
Cod					
dried, salted, boiled	100g	138	0	32.5	0.9
Fillets, baked, with butter added	100g	96	0	21.4	1.2
Fillets, baked, with butter added	50g portion	48	0	10.7	0.6
Fillets, baked, with butter added	120g portion	115	0	25.7	1.4
Fillets, baked, with butter added	175g portion	168	0	37.5	2.1
Fillets, poached in milk with butter added	100g	94	0	20.9	1.1
Fillets, poached in milk with butter added	50g portion	47	0	10.5	106
Fillets, poached in milk with butter added	120g portion	113	0	25.1	1.3
Fillets, poached in milk with butter added	175g portion	165	0	36.6	1.9
Fillets, raw	100g	76	0	17.4	0.7
in batter, fried in blended oil	100g	199	7.5	19.6	10.3

Specific	Amount	Kcals	Carb	Prot	Fat
in batter, fried in dripping	100g	199	7.5	19.6	10.3
in batter, fried in oil or dripping	120g portion	239	9.0	23.5	12.4
in batter, fried in oil or dripping	180g portion	358	13.5	35.3	18.5
in batter, fried in oil or dripping	225g portion	448	16.9	44.1	23.2
Steaks, frozen, raw,	100g	68	0	15.6	0.6
Crab					
boiled	100g	127	0	20.1	5.2
boiled crabmeat	1 tbsp [40g]	51	0	8.0	2.1
canned	100g	81	0	18.1	0.9
canned	1 small can [85g]	69	0	15.4	0.8
canned	1 large can [170g]	138	0	30.8	1.5
Dogfish					
in batter, fried	large portion [250g]	663	19.3	41.8	47.0
in batter, fried in blended oil	100g	265	7.7	16.7	18.8
in batter, fried in dripping	100g	265	7.7	16.7	18.8
in batter, fried in oil or dripping	small portion [150g]	400	11.6	25.1	28.2
in batter, fried in oil or dripping	medium portion [200g]	530	15.4	33.4	37.6
Fish fingers					
fried in blended oil	100g	233	17.2	13.5	12.7
fried in lard	100g	233	17.2	13.5	12.7
fried in oil or lard	1 fish finger [28g]	65	4.8	3.8	3.6
fried in oil or lard	1 jumbo-size fish finger [60g]	140	10.3	8.1	7.6
grilled	100g	214	19.3	15.1	9.0
grilled	1 fish finger [28g]	60	5.4	4.3	2.5

Calorie Values

Specific	Amount	Kcals	Carb	Prot	Fat
grilled	1 jumbo-size fish finger [60g]	128	11.6	9.1	5.4
Fish-based dish					
Fish pie, home-made	100g	105	12.3	8.0	3.0
Fish pie, home-made	250g portion	263	30.8	20	7.5
Kedgeree, home-made	100g	166	10.5	14.2	7.9
Kedgeree, home-made	300g portion	498	31.5	42.6	23.7
Fish-based product					
Fish cakes, fried	100g	188	15.1	9.1	10.5
Fish cakes, fried	1 fish cake [50g]	94	7.6	4.6	5.3
Fish paste	100g	169	3.7	15.3	10.4
Fish paste	medium jar [53g]	90	2.0	8.1	0.7
Fish paste	10g portion for bread	17	0.4	1.5	1.0
Taramasalata	100g	446	4.1	3.2	46.4
Taramasalata	1 tbsp [45g]	201	1.8	1.4	20.9
Haddock					
fillet, raw	100g	73	0	16.8	0.6
in breadcrumbs, fried in blended oil	100g	174	3.6	21.4	8.3
in breadcrumbs, fried in dripping	100g	174	3.6	21.4	8.3
in breadcrumbs, fried in oil or dripping	small portion [85g]	148	3.1	18.2	7.1
in breadcrumbs, fried in oil or dripping	medium portion [120g]	209	4.3	25.7	10.0
in breadcrumbs, fried in oil or dripping	large portion [170g]	296	6.1	36.4	12.1
middle cut, steamed	100g	98	0	22.8	0.8
middle cut, steamed	85g portion	83	0	19.4	0.7
smoked, steamed	100g	101	0	23.3	0.9

Specific	Amount	Kcals	Carb	Prot	Fat
smoked, steamed	85g portion	86	5.2	19.8	0.8
middle cut, steamed	100g	98	0	22.8	0.8
Halibut					
middle cut, steamed	85g portion	83	0	19.4	0.7
raw	100g	92	0	17.7	2.4
Herring					
fried in oatmeal	100g	234	1.5	23.1	15.1
fried in oatmeal	85g portion	199	1.3	19.6	12.8
fried in oatmeal	119g portion	278	1.8	27.5	18.0
grilled	100g	135	0	13.9	8.8
grilled	85g portion	115	0	11.8	7.5
grilled	119g portion	161	0	16.5	10.5
raw	100g	234	0	16.8	18.5
Kipper					
baked	100g	205	0	25.5	11.4
baked	125g portion	256	0	31.9	13.7
Lemon sole					
in breadcrumbs, fried	100g	216	9.3	16.1	13.0
in breadcrumbs, fried	small portion [90g]	194	8.4	14.5	11.7
in breadcrumbs, fried	medium portion [150g]	324	14.0	24.1	19.5
breadcrumbs, fried	large portion [220g]	475	20.5	35.4	28.6
raw	100g	81	0	17.1	1.4
steamed	100g	91	0	20.6	0.9
steamed	small portion [90g]	81	0	18.5	0.8
steamed	medium portion [150g]	137	0	30.9	1.4
steamed	large portion [220g]	200	0	45.3	2.0
Lobster					
boiled	100g	119	0	22.1	3.4

Calorie Values

Specific	Amount	Kcals	Carb	Prot	Fat
boiled	2 tbsp lobster meat[85g]	101	0	18.8	2.9
Mackerel					
fried	100g	188	0	21.5	11.3
fried	220g portion	414	0	47.3	28.3
raw	100g	223	0	19.0	16.3
smoked	100g	354	0	18.9	30.9
smoked	150g portion	531	0	28.4	46.4
Mussels					
boiled	100g	87	trace	17.2	2.0
boiled	1 mussel, no shell [7g]	6	trace	1.2	0.1
boiled	1 portion, no shells [40g]	35	trace	6.9	0.8
Pilchards					
in tomato sauce, canned	100g	126	0.7	18.8	5.4
in tomato sauce, canned	1 pilchard [55g]	69	0.4	10.3	3.0
in tomato sauce, canned	215g can	271	1.5	40.4	11.6
in batter, fried in dripping	100g	279	14.4	15.8	18.0
in batter, fried in oil or dripping	small portion [150g]	419	21.6	23.7	27.0
in batter, fried in oil or dripping	medium portion [200g]	558	28.8	31.6	36
in breadcrumbs, fried	100g	228	8.6	18.0	13.7
in breadcrumbs, fried	small portion [90g]	205	7.7	16.2	12.3
in breadcrumbs, fried	medium portion [150g]	342	12.9	27.0	20.6
in breadcrumbs, fried	large portion [200g]	456	17.2	36	27.4
raw	100g	91	0	17.9	2.2
steamed	100g	93	0	18.9	1.9

Specific	Amount	Kcals	Carb	Prot	Fat
steamed	small portion [75g]	70	0	14.2	1.4
steamed	medium portion [130g]	121	0	24.6	2.5
steamed	large portion [180g]	167	0	34.0	3.4
Prawns					
boiled	100g	107	0	22.6	1.8
boiled	1 prawn, no shell [3g]	3	0	0.7	0.1
boiled	average portion, [60g]	64	0	13.6	1.1
boiled for prawn cocktail	40g	43	0	9.0	0.8
Roe					
Cod, hard, in breadcrumbs, fried	100g	202	3.0	20.9	11.9
Cod, hard, in breadcrumbs, fried	116g portion	234	3.5	24.2	13.8
Herring, soft, rolled in flour and fried	100g	244	4.7	21.1	15.8
Herring, soft, rolled in flour and fried	85g portion	207	4.0	17.9	13.4
Saithe					
raw	100g	73	0	17.0	0.5
steamed	100g	99	0	23.3	0.6
steamed	130g portion	129	0	30.3	0.8
Salmon					
canned	100g	155	0	20.3	8.2
canned	portion for sandwich[40g]	62	0	8.1	3.3
raw	100g	182	0	18.4	12.0
smoked	100g	142	0	25.4	4.5
smoked	portion for sandwich[50g]	71	0	12.7	2.2

Specific	Amount	Kcals	Carb	Prot	Fat
steamed	100g	197	0	20.1	13.0
Sardines					
in oil, canned, drained	100g	217	0	23.7	13.6
in oil, canned, drained	1 sardine [25g]	54	0	5.9	3.4
in oil, canned, drained	portion for sandwich [40g]	109	0	11.9	6.8
in tomato sauce, canned	100g	177	0.5	17.8	11.6
in tomato sauce, canned	portion for sandwich [50g]	89	0.3	8.9	5.8
Scampi					
in breadcrumbs, fried	100g	316	28.9	12.2	17.6
in breadcrumbs, fried	1 piece [15g]	79	7.2	3.1	4.4
in breadcrumbs, fried	150g portion	474	43.4	18.3	26.4
Shrimps					
canned, drained	100g	94	0	20.8	1.2
canned, drained	average portion [60g]	56	0	12.5	0.7
frozen	100g	73	0	16.5	0.8
Skate					
in batter, fried	100g	199	4.9	17.9	12.1
in batter, fried	200g portion	398	9.8	35.8	24.2
Squid					
frozen, raw	100g	66	0	13.1	1.5
Trout					
Brown, steamed	100g	135	0	23.5	4.5
Brown, steamed	120g portion	162	0	28.2	5.4
Tuna					
in brine, canned, drained	100g	99	0	23.5	0.6
in brine, canned, drained	50g portion for sandwich	49	0	10.6	0.3
in brine, canned, drained	92g portion for salad	91	0	21.6	0.6
in oil, canned, drained	100g	189	0	27.1	9.0

Specific	Amount	Kcals	Carb	Prot	Fat
in oil, canned, drained	45g portion for sandwich	85	0	12.2	4.1
in oil, canned, drained	92g portion for salad	174	0	24.9	8.3
Whelks					
boiled, weighed with shell	100g	14	trace	2.8	0.3
Whitebait					
rolled in flour, fried	100g	525	5.3	19.5	47.5
rolled in flour, fried	1 whitebait [4g]	21	0.2	0.8	1.9
rolled in flour, fried	80g portion	420	4.2	15.6	38
Whiting					
in breadcrumbs, fried	100g	191	7.0	18.1	10.3
in breadcrumbs, fried	180g portion	344	12.6	32.6	18.5
steamed	100g	92	0	20.9	0.9
steamed	85g portion	78	0	17.8	0.8
Winkles					
boiled, weighed with shell	100g	14	trace	2.9	0.3

Desserts

Specific	Amount	Kcals	Carb	Prot	Fat
Blackcurrant pie					
home-made, pastry top and bottom	100g	262	34.5	3.1	13.3
home-made, pastry top and bottom	120g slice	314	41.4	3.7	16.0
Bread pudding					
home-made	100g	297	49.7	5.9	9.6
home-made	190g portion	564	94.4	11.2	18.2
Cheesecake					
frozen, with fruit	100g	242	33.0	5.7	10.6
frozen, with fruit	110g serving	266	36.3	6.3	11.7
individual, fruit purée topping	100g	274	32.4	5.8	13.5
individual, fruit purée topping	90g carton	247	29.2	5.2	12.2
Christmas pudding					
home-made	100g	291	49.5	4.6	9.7
retail	100g	329	56.3	3.0	11.8
Creamed Rice					
canned	100g	91	15.2	3.4	1.8
canned	425g can	387	64.6	14.5	7.7
canned	150g portion	137	22.8	5.1	2.7
Creamed Sago					
canned	100g	82	13.0	2.9	1.8
canned	425g can	349	55.3	12.3	7.7
canned	150g portion	123	19.5	4.4	2.7
Creamed Semolina					
canned	100g	84	13.2	3.6	1.9
canned	425g can	357	56.1	15.3	8.1

Specific	Amount	Kcals	Carb	Prot	Fat
canned	150g portion	126	19.8	5.4	2.9
Creme caramel					
individual	100g	109	20.6	3.0	2.2
individual	128g carton	140	26.4	3.8	2.8
Custard					
Chocolate-flavoured, powdered	100g, powder only	409	82.0	6.0	9.0
Chocolate-flavoured, powdered	1/4 pack serving, made with water	102	15.8	2.8	3.1
Devon, canned	425g can	434	67.2	11.0	13.2
Devon, canned	150g portion	153	23.7	4.2	4.7
home-made, made with skimmed milk	100g	79	16.8	3.8	0.1
home-made, made with skimmed milk	150g portion	119	25.2	5.7	0.2
home-made, made with whole milk	100g	117	16.6	3.7	4.5
home-made, made with whole milk	150g portion	176	24.9	5.6	6.7
low-fat, canned	100g	75	12.5	3.0	1.4
low-fat, canned	425g can	319	53.1	12.8	6.0
low-fat, canned	150g portion	113	18.8	4.5	2.1
Dessert topping					
Evaporated milk	100g	159	12.0	8.2	9.0
Evaporated milk	1 tbsp [15ml]	24	1.8	1.2	1.4
Tip Top	100g	112	9.0	4.8	6.3
Tip Top	50g serving	56	4.5	2.4	3.7
Frozen dessert					
Arctic roll	100g	200	33.3	4.1	6.6
Arctic roll	70g slice	140	23.3	2.9	4.6
Chocolate nut sundae, individual	100g	278	34.2	3.0	15.3
Chocolate nut sundae, individual	70g sundae	195	23.9	2.1	10.7

Calorie Values

Specific	Amount	Kcals	Carb	Prot	Fat
Viennetta	100g	272	27.6	3.8	16.4
Viennetta	50g slice	136	13.8	1.9	8.2
Frozen ice cream dessert, average	100g	227	22.8	3.3	14.2
Frozen ice cream dessert, average	45g slice	102	10.3	1.5	6.4
Fruit crumble					
Home-made	100g	198	34.0	2.0	6.9
Home-made	170g portion	337	57.8	3.4	11.7
Wholemeal, home-made	100g	193	31.7	2.6	7.1
Wholemeal, home-made	170g portion	328	53.9	4.4	12.1
Fruit pie					
pastry top and bottom	100g	262	34.5	3.1	13.3
pastry top and bottom	120g portion	314	41.4	3.7	16.0
Fruit pie filling					
Apple and blackberry, canned	100g	92	24.1	0.3	trace
Apple and blackberry, canned	385g can	354	92.8	1.2	trace
Black cherry, canned	100g	98	25.8	0.3	trace
Black cherry, canned	400g can	392	103.2	1.2	trace
Ice cream					
Choc ice	100g	277	28.1	3.5	17.5
Cornetto	100g	260	34.5	3.7	12.9
Cornetto	75g cone	195	25.8	2.8	9.7
Dairy, vanilla	100g	194	24.4	3.6	9.8
Dairy, vanilla	60g scoop	116	14.6	2.2	5.9
Flavoured	100g	179	24.7	3.5	8.0
Flavoured	60g scoop	107	14.8	2.1	4.8
Non-dairy, flavoured	100g	166	23.2	3.1	7.4
Non-dairy, flavoured	60g scoop	100	13.9	1.9	4.4
Non-dairy, vanilla	100g	178	23.1	3.2	8.7
Non-dairy, vanilla	60g scoop	107	13.9	1.9	5.2
Ice cream mix	100g	182	25.1	4.1	7.9

Specific	Amount	Kcals	Carb	Prot	Fat
Ice cream wafers	100g	342	78.8	10.1	0.7
Instant dessert powder					
Angel delight	100g, powder only	468	73.8	2.3	19.0
Angel delight	¼ pack serving, made with whole milk	128	13.9	2.9	5.8
Angel delight	¼ pack serving, madewith skimmed milk	104	13.9	2.9	3.2
Average, powder only	100g	391	60.1	2.4	17.3
Average, made with whole milk	100g	125	14.8	3.1	6.3
Average, made with whole milk	120g portion	150	17.8	3.7	7.6
Average, made with skimmed milk	100g	97	14.9	3.1	3.2
Average, made with skimmed milk	120g portion	116	17.9	3.7	3.8
Jelly					
Fruit-flavoured, before dilution	100g	280	69.7	4.7	trace
Lemon meringue pie					
Home-made	100g	319	45.9	4.5	14.4
Home-made	120g portion	383	55.1	5.4	17.3
Meringue					
Home-made	100g	379	95.4	5.3	trace
Home made	1 average [8g]	30	7.6	0.4	trace
Home-made, with cream	100g	376	40.0	3.3	23.6
Home-made, with cream	1 average [28g]	105	11.2	0.9	6.7
Mousse					
Chocolate, individual	100g	139	19.9	4.0	5.4
Chocolate, individual	60g carton	83	11.9	2.4	3.2
Fruit, individual	100g	137	18.0	4.5	5.7
Fruit, individual	60g carton	82	10.8	2.7	3.4

Calorie Values

Specific	Amount	Kcals	Carb	Prot	Fat
Pancakes					
Sweet, made with whole milk	100g	301	35.0	5.9	16.2
Sweet, made with whole milk	110g portion	331	38.5	6.5	17.8
Pie					
With pie filling	100g	273	34.6	3.2	14.5
With pie filling	120g portion	328	41.5	3.8	17.4
Rice Pudding					
Average, canned	100g	89	14.0	3.4	2.5
Average, canned	200g portion	178	28.0	6.8	5.0
Traditional, with sultanas and nutmeg	100g	101	17.1	3.3	2.6
Traditional, with sultanas and nutmeg	425g can	429	72.7	14.0	11.1
Traditional, with sultanas and nutmeg	150g portion	152	25.7	5.0	3.9
Sorbet					
Lemon, home-made	100g	131	34.2	0.9	trace
Lemon, home-made	60g scoop	79	20.5	0.5	trace
Sponge pudding					
Home-made	100g	340	45.3	5.8	16.3
Home-made	170g portion	578	77.0	9.9	27.7
Steamed sponge pudding					
Chocolate, with chocolate sauce, canned	100g	299	51.2	2.6	9.3
Chocolate, with chocolate sauce, canned	75g portion	225	38.4	2.0	7.0
Treacle, canned	100g	301	51.4	2.2	9.6
Treacle, canned	75g portion	226	38.6	1.7	7.2
with jam, canned	100g	299	49.8	2.6	9.9
with jam, canned	75g portion	224	37.4	2.0	7.4
Trifle					
Fruit cocktail, individual	100g	182	23.1	2.5	2.6

Specific	Amount	Kcals	Carb	Prot	Fat
Fruit cocktail, individual	113g carton	206	26.1	2.8	9.9
Home-made	100g	160	22.3	3.6	6.3
Home-made	170g portion	272	37.9	6.1	10.7
Home-made, with cream	100g	166	19.5	2.4	9.2
Home-made, with cream	170g portion	282	31.2	4.1	15.6
Milk chocolate, individual	100g	282	25.1	4.7	18.2
Milk chocolate, individual	105g carton	296	26.4	4.9	19.1
Raspberry, individual	100g	173	21.1	2.5	8.7
Raspberry, individual	113g carton	195	23.8	2.8	9.8
Yoghurt					
Greek, strained	100g	115	2.0	6.4	9.1
Greek, strained	150g serving	173	3.0	9.6	13.7
Low-fat, fruit	100g	90	17.9	4.1	0.7
Low-fat, fruit	150g pot	135	26.9	6.2	1.1
Low-fat, plain	100g	56	7.5	5.1	0.8
Low-fat, plain	150g pot	84	11.3	7.7	1.2
Very low-fat, fruit	100g	45	6.3	5.2	0.1
Very low-fat, fruit	150g pot	55	7.9	6.5	0.1
Whole milk, fruit	100g	105	15.7	5.1	2.8
Whole milk, fruit	150g pot	158	23.6	7.7	4.2
Whole milk, plain	100g	79	7.8	5.7	3.0
Whole milk, plain	150g pot	119	11.7	8.6	4.5

Sweet and Savoury Snacks

Specific	Amount	Kcals	Carb	Prot	Fat
Chocolate confectionery					
Aero	100g	522	58.3	7.7	28.7
Aero	1 standard bar	252	26.7	4.0	14.4
Boost	100g	515	60.1	6.2	27.6
Boost	1 bar [57g]	295	34.3	3.5	15.7
Bounty bar	100g	473	58.3	4.8	26.1
Bounty bar	1 mini bar [30g]	142	17.5	1.4	7.8
Caramac	100g	545	56.3	6.8	32.5
Caramac	1 bar [27g]	164	16.9	2.1	9.8
Chocolate cream	100g	425	72.6	2.7	13.7
Chocolate cream	1 bar [50g]	215	36.3	1.4	6.9
Chocolate, milk	100g	529	59.4	8.4	30.3
Chocolate, milk	50g bar	265	29.7	4.2	15.2
Chocolate, plain	100g	525	64.8	4.7	29.2
Chocolate, plain	50g bar	263	32.4	2.4	14.6
Chocolate, white	100g	529	58.3	8.0	30.9
Chocolate, white	50g bar	265	29.1	4.0	15.5
Chocolates [assorted]	100g	460	73.3	4.1	18.8
Creme egg	100g	385	58.0	4.1	16.8
Creme egg	1 egg [39g]	150	22.6	1.6	6.6
Crunchie	100g	460	72.7	4.6	19.1
Crunchie	1 bar [42g]	195	30.5	1.9	8.0
Dairy Milk	1 medium bar [54g]	285	30.7	4.3	15.9
Dairy Milk	100g	525	56.8	7.8	29.4
Flake	100g	505	58.4	8.2	28.5
Flake	1 bar	170	19.9	2.8	9.7
Fudge	1 bar [30g]	130	21.6	1.0	5.2
Fudge	100g	420	72.1	3.4	17.2

Specific	Amount	Kcals	Carb	Prot	Fat
Kit Kat	100g	499	60.5	8.2	26.6
Kit Kat	2-finger bar [20g]	100	12.1	1.6	5.3
Kit Kat	4 finger bar [50g]	250	30	0.8	2.7
Mars Bar	100g	441	66.5	5.3	18.9
Mars Bar	1 mini bar [20g]	88	13.3	1.1	3.8
Mars Bar	[68g]	300	9.0	0.7	2.6
Milky Bar	100g	549	55.6	8.4	32.5
Milky Bar	1 medium bar [20g]	110	11.1	1.7	6.4
Milky Way	100g	397	63.4	4.4	15.8
Milky Way	1 bar [55g]	218	34.8	2.4	8.7
Smarties	100g	456	73.9	5.4	17.5
Smarties	1 tube [36g]	164	26.6	1.9	6.3
Topic	100g	497	56.7	7.4	26.7
Topic	1 bar [54g]	268	30.6	4.0	14.4
Turkish Delight	100g	370	69.0	1.6	7.7
Turkish Delight	1 bar [51g]	190	37.8	0.8	3.9
Twirl	100g	525	55.9	8.1	30.1
Twirl	1 finger	115	12.3	1.8	6.6
Twix	100g	480	63.2	5.6	24.5
Twix	50g bar	240	31.6	2.8	12.3

Non-chocolate Confectionery

Specific	Amount	Kcals	Carb	Prot	Fat
Boiled sweets	100g	327	87.3	trace	trace
Fruit Gums	100g	172	44.8	1.0	0
Fruit Gums	1 tube [33g]	57	14.8	0.3	0
Liquorice Allsorts	1 small bag [56g]	175	41.5	2.2	1.2
Liquorice Allsorts	100g	313	74.1	3.9	2.2
Starburst	100g	411	85.3	0.3	7.6
Starburst	1 pack [56g]	230	47.7	0.2	4.3
Pastilles, assorted	100g	253	61.9	5.2	0
Peppermints, assorted	100g	392	102.2	0.5	0.7

Calorie Values

Specific	Amount	Kcals	Carb	Prot	Fat
Popcorn, candied	100g	592	77.6	2.1	20.0
Popcorn, plain	100g	480	48.6	6.2	42.8
Skittles	100g	383	91.5	0.3	4.3
Skittles	1 pack [60g]	230	54.9	0.2	2.6
Toffees, mixed	100g	430	71.1	2.1	17.2
Turkish Delight	100g	295	77.9	0.6	0
Turkish Delight	50g bar	198	38.9	0.3	0
Savoury Snacks					
Bombay mix	100g	503	35.1	18.8	32.9
Cheddars	100g	534	52.9	11.3	30.2
Corn snacks	100g	519	54.3	7.0	31.9
Peanuts and raisins	100g	435	37.5	15.3	26.0
Potato crisps, assorted	100g	546	49.3	5.6	37.6
Potato crisps, assorted	28g bag	153	13.8	1.6	10.5
Potato crisps, low-fat, assorted	100g	456	63.0	6.6	21.5
Potato crisps, low-fat, assorted	28g bag	128	17.6	1.8	6.0
Potato Hoops	100g	523	58.5	3.9	32.0
Skips [KP]	100g	512	59.8	4.2	28.4
Skips [KP]	18g bag	92	10.8	0.8	5.1
Tortilla Chips	100g	459	60.1	7.6	22.6
Trail Mix	100g	432	37.2	9.1	28.5
Twiglets	100g	383	62.0	11.3	11.7
Wotsits	100g	545	52.4	9.4	33.1
Wotsits	21g bag	115	11.0	2.0	7.0

Jams and Preserves

Specific	Amount	Kcals	Carb	Prot	Fat
Preserves					
Jam, fruit	100g	261	69.0	0.6	0
Jam, fruit	15g portion	39	10.4	0.1	0
Jam, fruit	1 tsp [18g]	47	12.4	0.1	0
Jam, stone fruit	100g	261	69.3	0.4	0
Jam, stone fruit	15g portion	39	10.4	0.1	0
Jam, stone fruit	1 tsp [18g]	47	12.5	0.1	0
Jam, reduced sugar	100g	123	31.9	0.5	0
Jam, reduced sugar	15g portion	18	4.8	0.1	0
Jam, reduced sugar	1 tsp [18g]	22	5.7	0.1	0
Lemon curd	100g	283	62.7	0.6	5.1
Lemon curd	15g portion	42	9.4	0.1	0.8
Lemon curd	1 tsp [18g]	51	11.3	0.1	0.9
Marmalade	100g	261	69.5	0.1	0
Marmalade	15g portion	39	10.4	trace	0
Marmalade	1 tsp [18g]	47	12.5	trace	0
Mincemeat	100g	274	62.1	0.6	4.3
Spread					
Chocolate nut	100g	549	60.5	6.2	33.0
Chocolate nut	20g portion	110	12.1	1.2	6.6
Chocolate nut	1 tsp [16g]	88	9.7	1.0	5.3
Honey	100g	288	76.4	0.4	0
Honey	20g portion	58	15.3	0.1	0
Honey	1 tsp [17g]	49	13.0	0.1	0
Honey & comb	100g	281	74.4	0.6	4.6
Honey & comb	20g portion	56	14.9	0.1	0.9
Sugar					
Demerara	100g	394	104.5	0.5	0
Demerara	1 tsp [20g]	79	20.9	0.1	0

Calorie Values

Specific	Amount	Kcals	Carb	Prot	Fat
Demerara	1 level tsp [4g]	16	4.2	trace	0
Demerara	7g sachet	28	7.3	trace	0
Glucose liquid	100g	318	84.7	trace	0
White	100g	394	105.0	trace	0
White	1 tbsp [20g]	79	21.0	trace	0
White	1 level tsp [4g]	16	4.2	trace	0
White	1 cube [5g]	20	5.3	trace	0
Syrup, golden	100g	298	79.0	0.3	0
Treacle, black	100g	257	67.2	1.2	0

Soups, Chutneys and Miscellaneous

Specific	Amount	Kcals	Carb	Prot	Fat
Chutney					
Apple	100g	201	52.2	0.9	0.2
Apple	40g portion	80	20.9	0.4	0.1
Apple	1 tsp [15g]	30	7.8	0.1	trace
Mango	100g	285	49.5	0.4	10.9
Mango	40g portion	114	19.8	0.2	4.4
Mango	1 tsp [15g]	43	7.4	0.1	1.6
Tomato	100g	161	40.9	1.2	0.4
Tomato	40g portion	64	16.4	0.5	0.2
Tomato	1 tsp [15g]	24	6.1	0.2	0.1
Miscellaneous					
Baking powder	100g	163	37.8	5.2	trace
Baking powder	1 level tsp	7	1.5	0.2	trace
Bovril	100g	169	2.9	38.0	0.7
Bovril	3g portion	5	0.1	1.1	trace
Bovril	1 level tsp [9g]	15	0.3	3.4	trace
Gelatine	100g	338	0	84	0
Gravy granules, made with water	100g	462	40.6	4.4	32.5
Gravy granules, made with water	medium portion [70g]	323	28.4	3.1	22.8
Marmite	100g	172	1.8	39.7	0.7
Marmite	3g portion	5	0.1	1.2	trace
Marmite	1 level tsp [9g]	15	0.2	3.6	0.1
Mustard, smooth	100g	139	9.7	7.1	8.2
Mustard smooth	1 level tsp [8g]	11	0.8	0.6	0.7
Mustard, wholegrain	100g	140	4.2	8.2	10.2
Mustard, wholegrain	1 level tsp	11	0.3	0.7	0.8
Oxo cubes	100g	229	12.0	38.3	3.4

Calorie Values

Specific	Amount	Kcals	Carb	Prot	Fat
Oxo cubes	1 cube [7g]	16	0.8	2.7	0.2
Salt	100g	0	0	0	0
Salt	1 tsp	0	0	0	0
Vinegar	100g	4	0.6	0.4	0
Vinegar	1 tbsp [15g]	1	0.1	0.1	0
Yeast, baker's compressed	100g	5	1.1	11.4	0.4
Yeast, dried	100g	169	3.5	35.6	1.5
Pickle					
Sweet	100g	134	34.4	0.6	0.3
Sweet	40g portion	54	13.8	0.2	0.1
Sweet	1 tsp [15g]	20	5.2	trace	trace
Salad dressing					
French dressing	100g	649	0.1	0.3	72.1
French dressing	15g portion	97	trace	trace	10.8
Mayonnaise	100g	691	1.7	1.1	75.6
Mayonnaise	30g portion	207	0.5	0.3	22.7
Mayonnaise	1 tbsp [33g]	68	0.2	0.1	7.5
Salad cream	100g	348	16.7	1.5	31.0
Salad cream	30g portion	104	5.0	0.5	9.3
Salad cream, reduced calorie	100g	194	9.4	1.0	17.2
Salad cream, reduced calorie	30g portion	58	2.8	0.3	5.2
Sauce					
Barbecue	100g	75	12.2	1.8	1.8
Barbecue sauce	30g portion	23	3.7	0.5	0.5
Bread sauce, made with semi-skimmed milk	100g	93	12.8	4.3	3.1
Bread sauce, made with semi-skimmed milk	45g portion	42	5.8	1.9	1.4
Bread sauce, made with whole milk	100g	110	12.6	4.2	5.1
Bread sauce, made with whole milk	45g portion	50	5.7	9.2	11.2

Specific	Amount	Kcals	Carb	Prot	Fat
Brown sauce, bottled	100g	99	25.2	1.1	0
Brown sauce, bottled	30g portion	30	7.6	0.3	0
Cheese sauce, made with semi-skimmed milk	100g	179	9.1	8.1	12.6
Cheese sauce, made with semi-skimmed milk	medium portion [60g]	107	5.5	4.9	7.6
Cheese sauce, made with whole milk	100g	197	8.0	14.6	
Cheese sauce, made with whole milk	medium portion [60g]	118	5.4	4.8	8.7
Cheese sauce, packet mix, made with semi-skimmed milk	100g	90	9.5	5.4	3.8
Cheese sauce, packet mix, made with semi-skimmed milk	medium portion [60g]	54	5.7	3.2	2.3
Cheese sauce, packet mix, made with whole milk	100g	110	9.3	5.3	6.1
Cheese sauce, packet mix, made with whole milk	medium portion [60g]	66	5.6	3.2	3.7
Cook-in sauces, canned, average	100g	43	8.3	1.1	0.8
Cook-in sauces, canned, average	115g portion	49	9.5	1.3	0.9
Curry sauce, canned	100g	78	7.1	1.5	5.0
Curry sauce, canned	115g portion	90	8.2	1.7	5.8
Horseradish sauce	100g	153	17.9	2.5	8.4
Horseradish sauce	15g portion	23	2.7	0.4	1.3
Mint sauce	100g	87	21.5	1.6	trace
Mint sauce	10g portion	9	2.2	0.2	trace

Calorie Values

Specific	Amount	Kcals	Carb	Prot	Fat
Onion sauce, made with semi-skimmed milk	100g	86	8.4	2.9	5.0
Onion sauce, made with semi-skimmed milk	medium portion [60g]	52	5.0	1.7	3.0
Onion sauce, made with whole milk	100g	99	8.3	2.8	6.5
Onion sauce, made with whole milk	medium portion [60g]	60	5.0	1.7	3.9
Pasta sauce, tomato based	100g	47	6.9	2.0	1.5
Pasta sauce, tomato base	90g portion	42	6.2	1.8	1.4
Soy sauce	100g	64	8.3	8.7	0
Soy sauce	1 tsp [5g]	3	0.4	0.4	0
Tomato ketchup	100g	98	24.0	2.1	trace
Tomato ketchup	30g portion	29	7.2	0.6	trace
Tomato sauce, home-made	100g	89	8.6	2.2	5.5
Tomato sauce, home-made	30g portion	27	2.6	0.7	1.7
White sauce, savoury, made with semi-skimmed milk	100g	128	11.1	4.2	7.8
White sauce, savoury, made with semi-skimmed milk	medium portion [60g]	77	6.6	2.5	4.7
White sauce, savoury, made withwhole milk	100g	150	10.9	4.1	10.3
White sauce, savoury, made with whole milk	medium portion [60g]	90	6.5	2.5	6.2
White sauce, sweet, made withsemi-skimmed milk	100g	150	18.8	3.9	7.2
White sauce, sweet, made withsemi-skimmed milk	medium portion [60g]	90	11.3	2.3	4.3

Soups, Chutneys and Miscellaneous

Specific	Amount	Kcals	Carb	Prot	Fat
White sauce, sweet, made with whole milk	100g	170	18.6	3.8	9.5
White sauce, sweet, made with whole milk	medium portion [60g]	102	11.2	2.3	5.7
Soup					
Chicken noodle, dried, cooked	100g	20	3.7	0.8	0.3
Chicken noodle, dried, cooked	medium portion [220g]	44	8.1	1.8	0.7
Cream of chicken, canned	100g	58	4.5	1.7	3.8
Cream of chicken, canned	medium portion [220g]	128	9.9	3.7	8.4
Cream of chicken, condensed, canned	100g	98	6.0	2.6	7.2
Cream of chicken, condensed, diluted	100g	49	3.0	1.3	3.6
Cream of chicken, condensed, diluted	medium portion [220g]	108	6.6	2.9	7.9
Cream of mushroom soup, canned	100g	53	3.9	1.1	3.8
Cream of mushroom, canned	medium portion [220g]	117	8.6	2.4	8.4
Cream of tomato, canned	100g	55	5.9	0.8	3.3
Cream of tomato, canned	medium portion [220g]	121	13.0	1.8	7.3
Cream of tomato, condensed, canned	100g	123	14.6	1.7	6.8
Cream of tomato, condensed, diluted	100g	62	7.3	0.9	3.4
Cream of tomato, condensed, diluted	medium portion [220g]	136	16.1	2.0	7.5

Calorie Values

Specific	Amount	Kcals	Carb	Prot	Fat
Instant soup powder, average, made with water, cooked	100g	64	10.5	1.1	2.3
Instant soup powder, average, made with water,cooked	medium portion [220g]	141	23	2.4	5.1
Lentil, home-made	100g	99	12.7	4.4	3.8
Lentil, home-made	medium portion [220g]	218	27.9	9.7	8.4
Low-calorie, average, canned	100g	20	4.0	0.9	0.2
Low-calorie, average, canned	medium portion [220g]	44	8.8	2.0	0.4
Minestrone, dried,cooked	100g	298	47.6	10.1	8.8
Minestrone, dried,cooked	medium portion [220g]	656	104.7	22.2	19.4
Oxtail, canned	100g	44	5.1	2.4	1.7
Oxtail, canned	medium portion [220g]	97	11.2	5.3	3.7
Oxtail, dried, cooked	100g	27	3.9	1.4	0.8
Oxtail, dried, cooked	medium portion [220g]	59	8.6	3.1	1.8
Tomato, dried, cooked	100g	31	6.3	0.6	0.5
Tomato, dried, cooked	medium portion [220g]	68	13.9	1.3	1.1
Vegetable, canned,cooked	100g	37	6.7	1.5	0.7
Vegetable, canned,cooked	medium portion [220g]	81	14.7	3.3	1.5

Drinks

Specific	Amount	Kcals	Carb	Prot	Fat
Bournvita					
Semi-skimmed milk	100g	58	7.8	3.5	1.6
Semi-skimmed milk	1 mug [260g]	151	20.3	9.1	4.2
Whole milk	100g	76	7.6	3.4	3.8
Whole milk	1 mug [260g]	198	19.8	8.9	9.9
Powder	100g	341	79.0	7.7	1.5
Powder	portion [8g]	27	6.3	0.6	0.1
Build-up					
Semi-skimmed milk	100g	80	11.9	5.7	1.5
Semi-skimmed milk	1 mug [260g]	208	30.9	14.8	3.9
Whole milk	100g	98	11.7	5.6	3.6
Whole milk	1 mug [260g]	255	30.4	14.6	9.4
Carbonated drink					
Coca-cola	100g	36	10.5	trace	0
Coca-cola	can [330g]	119	5.0	trace	0
Lemonade, bottled	100g	21	5.6	trace	0
Lemonade, bottled	1 glass [200g]	42	11.2	trace	0
Lucozade, bottled	100g	67	18.0	trace	0
Lucozade, bottled	1 glass [200g]	134	36.0	trace	0
Cocoa					
Semi-skimmed milk	100g	57	7.0	3.5	1.9
Semi-skimmed milk	1 mug [260g]	148	18.2	22.9	4.9
Whole milk	100g	76	6.8	3.4	4.2
Whole milk	1 mug [260g]	198	17.7	8.8	10.9
Powder	100g	312	11.5	18.5	21.7
Powder	1 tsp [6g]	19	0.7	1.1	1.3
Coffee					
Instant, powder	100g	11.0	14.6	0	
Instant, powder	1 tsp [2g]	9	0.2	0.3	0

Calorie Values

Specific	Amount	Kcals	Carb	Prot	Fat
Instant, 30g of whole milk	1 mug	22	1.6	1.3	1.2
Instant, without milk or sugar	1 mug [260g]	2	0.2	0.3	0
Coffeemate					
Powder	100g	540	57.3	2.7	34.9
Powder	portion [6g]	32	3.4	0.2	2.1
Complan					
Sweet, water	100g	96	13.4	4.5	3.1
Sweet, water	1 mug [260g]	250	34.8	11.7	8.1
Sweet, whole milk	100g	145	16.9	6.9	6.1
Sweet, whole milk	1 mug [260g]	377	43.9	17.9	15.9
Sweet, powder	100g	430	57.9	20.0	14.0
Cordial					
Lime juice cordial, undiluted	100g	112	29.8	0.1	0
Lime juice cordial, undiluted	1 glass [40g]	45	11.9	trace	0
Rosehip syrup, undiluted	100g	232	4.8	trace	0
Rosehip syrup, undiluted	1 glass [40g]	93	1.9	trace	0
Drinking chocolate					
Semi-skimmed milk	100g	71	10.8	3.5	1.9
Semi-skimmed milk	1 mug [260g]	185	28.1	9.1	4.9
Whole milk	100g	90	10.6	3.4	4.1
Whole milk	1 mug [260g]	234	27.6	8.8	10.7
Powder	100g	366	77.4	5.5	6.0
Powder	1 mug [18g]	66	13.9	1.0	1.1
Horlicks					
Instant, water	100g	51	10.1	2.4	0.5
Instant, water	1 mug [260g]	133	26.6	6.2	1.3
Semi-skimmed milk	100g	81	12.9	4.3	1.9
Semi-skimmed milk	1 mug [260g]	211	33.5	11.2	4.9
Whole milk	100g	99	12.7	4.2	3.9
Whole milk	1 mug [260g]	257	33.0	10.9	10.1
Powder	100g	378	78.0	12.4	4.0

Specific	Amount	Kcals	Carb	Prot	Fat
Powder	portion [25g]	95	19.5	0.4	1.0
Powder, low-fat, instant	portion [32g]	119	23.3	5.6	1.1
Powder, low-fat, instant	100g	373	72.9	17.4	3.3
Juice					
Apple juice, unsweetened	100g	38	9.9	0.1	0.1
Apple juice, unsweetened	1 glass [200g]	76	328	0.2	0.2
Grape juice, unsweetened	100g	46	11.7	0.3	0.1
Grape juice, unsweetened	1 glass [200g]	92	23.4	0.6	0.2
Grapefruit juice, unsweetened	100g	33	8.3	0.4	0.1
Grapefruit juice, unsweetened	1 glass [200g]	66	16.6	0.8	0.2
Lemon juice, unsweetened	100g	7	1.6	0.3	trace
Lemon juice, unsweetened	1 tbsp [15g]	1	0.2	trace	trace
Orange juice, unsweetened	100g	36	8.8	0.5	0.1
Orange juice, unsweetened	1 glass [200g]	72	17.6	1.0	0.2
Pineapple juice, unsweetened	100g	41	10.5	0.3	0.1
Pineapple juice, unsweetened	1 glass [200g]	82	21.0	0.6	0.2
Tomato juice	100g	14	3.0	0.8	trace
Tomato juice	1 glass [200g]	28	6.0	1.6	trace
Milk shake					
Semi-skimmed milk	1 glass [200g]	138	22.6	6.4	3.2
Semi-skimmed milk	100g	69	11.3	3.2	1.6
Whole milk	100g	87	11.1	3.1	3.7
Whole milk	1 glass [200g]	174	22.2	6.2	7.4
Powder	100g	388	98.3	1.3	1.6
Powder	portion [15g]	58	14.7	0.2	0.2
Thick, take-away	100g	90	13.2	2.9	3.2

Calorie Values

Specific	Amount	Kcals	Carb	Prot	Fat
Thick, take-away	portion [300g]	270	39.6	8.7	9.6
Ovaltine					
Semi-skimmed milk	100g	79	13.0	3.9	1.7
Semi-skimmed milk	1 mug [260g]	205	33.8	10.1	4.4
Whole milk	100g	97	12.9	3.8	3.8
Whole milk	1 mug [260g]	252	4.9	9.9	9.9
Powder	100g	358	79.4	9.0	2.7
Powder	portion [25g]	90	19.9	2.3	0.7
Squash					
Orange drink, undiluted	100g	107	28.5	trace	0
Orange drink, undiluted	1 glass [40g]	43	11.4	trace	0
Ribena	100g	228	60.8	0.1	0
Ribena	1 glass [40g]	91	24.3	trace	0
Tea					
No milk or sugar	100g	trace	trace	0.1	trace
No milk or sugar	1 cup [200g]	trace	trace	0.2	trace
With 30g of whole milk	1 cup [200g]	20	1.4	1.2	1.2

Alcoholic Drinks

Specific	Amount	Kcals	Carb	Prot	Fat
Ale					
Bottled, brown	100ml	28	3	trace	nil
Bottled, brown	1 pt	159	17	trace	nil
Bottled, pale	100ml	32	2	trace	nil
Bottled, pale	1 pt	182	11.4	trace	nil
Strong	100ml	72	6.1	trace	nil
Strong	1 pt	409	34.6	trace	nil
Beer					
Bitter, canned	100ml	32	2.3	trace	nil
Bitter, canned	1 pt	182	13.1	trace	nil
Bitter, draught	100ml	32	2.3	trace	nil
Bitter, draught	1 pt	182	13.1	trace	nil
Bitter, keg	100ml	31	2.3	trace	nil
Bitter, keg	1 pt	177	13.1	trace	nil
Mild, draught	100ml	25	1.6	trace	nil
Mild, draught	1 pt	142	9.1	trace	nil
Stout	100ml	37	4.2	trace	nil
Stout	1 pt	210	23.5	trace	nil
Stout, extra	100ml	39	2.1	trace	nil
Stout, extra	1 pt	222	11.9	trace	nil
Cider					
Dry	100ml	36	2.6	trace	nil
Dry	1 pt	204	14.8	trace	nil
Sweet	100ml	42	4.3	trace	nil
Sweet	1 pt	238	24.4	trace	nil
Vintage	100ml	101	7.3	trace	nil
Vintage	1 pt	573	41.5	trace	nil
Fortified Wine					
Port	30ml	47	3.6	trace	nil

Calorie Values

Specific	Amount	Kcals	Carb	Prot	Fat
Sherry, dry	30ml	35	0.5	trace	nil
Sherry, medium	30ml	35	1.0	trace	nil
Sherry, sweet	30ml	43	2	trace	nil
Lager					
Bottled	100ml	29	1.5	trace	nil
Bottled	1 pt	165	8.5	trace	nil
Spirits					
Brandy, 40% proof	30ml	65	trace	trace	nil
Gin, 40% proof	30ml	65	trace	trace	nil
Rum, 40% proof	30ml	65	trace	trace	nil
Vodka, 40% proof	30ml	65	trace	trace	nil
Whisky, 40% proof	30ml	65	trace	trace	nil
Wine					
Red	100ml	68	0.3	trace	nil
Red	1 bottle [750ml]	510	2.3	trace	nil
Red	1 glass [120ml]	82	0.4	trace	nil
Rose, medium	100ml	71	2.5	trace	nil
Rose, medium	1bottle [750ml]	533	18.8	trace	nil
Rose, medium	1 glass [120ml]	853	3.0	trace	nil
White, dry	100ml	66	0.6	trace	nil
White, dry	1 bottle [750ml]	495	4.5	trace	nil
White, dry	1 glass [120ml]	79	0.7	trace	nil
White, medium	100ml	75	3.4	trace	nil
White, medium	1 bottle [750ml]	563	25.5	trace	nil
White, medium	1 glass [120ml]	90	4.1	trace	nil
White, sparkling	100ml	76	1.4	trace	nil
White, sparkling	1 bottle [750ml]	570	10.5	trace	nil
White, sparkling	1 glass [120ml]	91	1.7	trace	nil
White, sweet	100ml	94	5.9	trace	nil
White, sweet	1 bottle [750ml]	705	44.3	trace	nil
White, sweet	1 glass [120ml]	113	53.2	trace	nil

Appendix
Vitamins and Minerals

Symbols used in the text:

μg	microgram
μl^{-1}	micrograms per litre
μmol	micromole
IU	international unit

Introduction

Human health is governed by two critical factors—the inherited genetic characteristics from our parents and our environment and living habits. We can do nothing to alter our genetic inheritance, but we can benefit our health by choosing the correct lifestyle and living habits. This should mean we lower our risks of developing certain diseases, e.g. cancer, and extend our life-span and improve our quality of life.

Our health can be influenced by a huge range of factors—eating habits, alcohol, exercise, coffee, occupation, food quality, tobacco, sleep and stress. This list is not a complete one, but it can be seen how many factors relate to the food and drink we consume. Much of the food eaten today is in a processed form, which is convenient but may be lacking in essential nutrients, vitamins and minerals. In a healthy diet, we should consume a balance of carbohydrates, proteins, fats, fibre, vegetables and fruit. Carbohydrates are starches and sugars found in foodstuffs, and they are the body's main source of energy. Health authorities recommend that we eat more starchy food, such as potatoes, bread, rice, pasta and maize, and cut down our intake of sugars, particularly refined sugars found in cakes, biscuits, chocolate, etc. Sugars do occur naturally in foods like milk and fruit but refined sugar has no nutrient value, it just has 'empty' calories. Proteins are required for the growth and repair of our body cells. Once digested, proteins break down into amino acids, which go to form new protein components inside cells. Humans need eight essential amino acids from proteins in our diet as they cannot be made inside our bodies. They include valine, leucine, methionine and tryptophan, the last of which can be converted into vitamin B_3 (niacin) in humans. Protein can be plant or animal in origin, but some of the plant protein sources may lack some of the essential amino acids. Protein is found in meat, fish, eggs, dairy products, whole-grain cereals, pasta, beans, maize, peas and nuts.

We also need fats in our diet. When digested, fats release fatty acids, which are needed to build and repair cells and to act as chemical messengers to activate body functions. Fat is also used as an energy source. There are two types of fat: saturated and unsaturated. Saturated fats are hard at room temperature as they have a structure with as many hydrogen atoms as possible in it (hence saturated fat). They are found in dairy foods, beef, lamb, pork, meat products, milk, eggs, cakes, biscuits, chocolate and some vegetable oils, e.g. coconut and palm oil. Saturated fats in our diet may be used to produce cholesterol in the liver. Many people have heard of cholesterol as it may be linked to heart attacks or stroke. Cholesterol is essential for many body functions, including making hormones and reproduction.

There are two forms of cholesterol: low-density lipoprotein (LDL) and high density lipoprotein (HDL). LDL-cholesterol is the 'bad' form of the fat as it removes some LDL-cholesterol to the cells for use but leaves any excess in the bloodstream where it can gradually block the arteries, reducing blood flow and increasing the risks of heart attack or strokes. HDL-cholesterol acts to remove this excess fat from the bloodstream and so reduces the chances of blocked arteries and circulatory problems.

Unsaturated fats are fats that do not have their full complement of hydrogen atoms in their structure. There are two types: polyunsaturated fats, which are found in fish, chicken, soft margarines labelled high in polyunsaturates, and very low fat spreads made with unsaturated oils. They are also found in vegetable oils like safflower, corn or sunflower oil and soya bean oil. Until recently, polyunsaturated fats were considered good for us and not damaging in the same way as saturated fats are. Now it appears that polyunsaturated fats are attacked by oxygen-free radicals, making them oxidized and rancid. This could lead to damage to the artery walls in our body. Instead, consumption of monounsaturated fats is encouraged. These are found in olive oil, rape-seed oil, peanut oil, peanuts, avocado and olives. There are also several monounsaturated fat spreads on the market, but care has to be taken as they may have been hardened into a solid by the addition of hydrogenated oil. This oil contains trans-fatty acids, which act similarly to saturated fats in our bloodstream. We should avoid spreads containing these fatty acids and some spreads now promote the reduced levels of trans-fatty acids in their product. Hydrogenated vegetable fat and oil is also found in biscuits, crisps, cakes and cereals.

Our diet should contain a good balance of carbohydrate, protein, vegetables, fruit, fibre and fats. A diet with not more than 30 per cent fat is recommended, with only a third of that saturated fat. We should eat more monounsaturated than polyunsaturated fats as well. This would decrease the levels of triglyceride fats in our blood (which come from our diet) and so reduce the risks of death from heart disease, particularly in women.

Fibre is the part of vegetable, fruits and unrefined cereal grains that we cannot digest. Like fats, there are two types, soluble and insoluble. Soluble fibre is found in fruit, vegetables, beans and oats, and in the body it modifies the absorption of fats and lowers the levels of blood cholesterol. Insoluble fibre acts to add bulk to the faeces, so helping its movement through the intestines and preventing constipation. It speeds up the time taken for digested food to move through the large intestine, so reducing exposure of the intestine to any harmful toxins or carcinogens present in our food. This is thought to help protect against cancer of the colon. Fibre can also stabilize sugar absorption, which is important for diabetics. Dietary fibre, however, may absorb some medicines and reduce their speed of absorption into the body. We should aim to eat 25g (1oz) of fibre every day.

Government health authorities now recommend we eat at least five portions of fruit and vegetables a day. Many of the chemicals that give the fruit or vegetables their colour are protective factors, and they work with vitamins in our food to stimulate the immune system. These protective factors are found in a massive range of fruit and vegetables, including cabbage, broccoli, carrots, strawberries, turnips, cauliflower, onions, green peppers, pineapples and tomatoes.

Another common item in our diet about which there is great debate is coffee. Conflicting studies have shown both protective and harmful effects from drinking coffee. The caffeine can overstimulate some people, causing agitation. Caffeine can also be addictive, even if drunk at only moderate levels. A study where people who drank 2–3 cups of coffee a day stopped doing so resulted in some people having headaches, anxiety and depression. It is probably wise to cut down on the levels of caffeine taken in drinks or to replace it with coffee substitutes or herbal teas, which do not contain caffeine. Tea also contains caffeine, so its intake should be limited as well.

The vegetarian diet

A vegetarian diet requires the same balance of carbohydrate, protein, fats, fibre but with a higher emphasis on vegetables and fruit. The degree to which a diet is vegetarian varies, as some people exclude meat, poultry and fish but others do leave fish in their diets. A lacto-vegetarian excludes eggs but eats milk and milk products, while an ovo-vegetarian eats both eggs and milk products. This is along with the normal vegetarian diet of vegetables, fruit, beans, grains, nuts, sprouts and mushrooms. A vegan does not eat any product from the animal kingdom. The risk of malnutrition and vitamin or mineral deficiency is not as great as once thought with a vegetarian diet. Adequate levels of essential amino acids can be obtained from plant proteins, eggs, milk and from pulses. Vitamins such as cyanocobalamin (B_{12}) are not present in plants, so a vegan may become deficient in this nutrient. Vitamin B_{12} is present in milk, so lacto- or ovo-vegetarians are not at risk from lack of vitamins B_{12}, D or B_2 (riboflavin). Vitamin-fortified soya milk contains vitamins D, B_{12} and B_2, but since this is not consumed by vegans they may require supplements. Calcium may also be lacking in vegans although it is present in tofu, flour, corn meal, sesame seeds, molasses and almond or filbert nuts. Vegetarians are commonly thought to be anaemic and lacking in iron as the best source of iron is meat. Iron from vegetables is harder to absorb into the body, but this can be helped by eating vitamin C-rich fruits, which aid absorption of iron.

Soya beans or their products, e.g. milk, tofu, often replace eggs, milk and meat in vegetarian diets, and they contain protein, vitamin E, iron, calcium, magnesium and phosphorus. Vegetarians need to have a balanced diet. If not they may develop deficiencies of selenium, copper, zinc, magnesium and lack sufficient dietary fibre. Children are at particular risk of too little vitamin D and calcium if they have a vegetarian diet. Women should take supplements of vitamin B_{12} as deficiency can cause irreversible nerve and brain damage. This is a particular risk when a woman is pregnant or breast-feeding, as the infant can deplete her stores of B_{12} and the child can suffer damage too if B_{12} is lacking. All vegan mothers are recommended to eat products fortified with vitamin B_{12} or to take B_{12} supplements.

The digestive process

The human digestive system is made up of the alimentary canal and several glands that secrete digestive juices into it. Food enters the mouth and is chewed so the teeth break down the food, increasing its surface area and making it easier to swallow. Saliva is produced from the salivary glands, and this lubricates the food and delivers a digestive enzyme to the mouth. This enzyme, called salivary amylase, breaks down starch into a smaller sugar called maltose. Saliva also helps to neutralize acid in the mouth and kill most of the bacteria present in the oral cavity. The food is swallowed and 5–10 seconds later it has moved down the oesophagus and entered the stomach. This organ is large enough to store a whole meal, so humans do not have to eat constantly in the same way as some animals do. The stomach lining produces gastric juice, which has an acidic pH of around 2. This acid kills any bacteria swallowed with the food and helps to break down the intercellular connections in meat or plants. An enzyme called pepsin is also found in gastric juice, and it breaks down proteins into smaller polypeptide units.

The contents of the stomach are mixed by the churning action of the muscles, and a nutrient mixture called acid chyme is produced. Despite public belief, little digestion of the food occurs in the stomach. Over a period of two to six hours after a meal, the acid chyme is released into the small intestine. Here digestive juices from the intestinal wall, pancreas, liver and gall bladder are mixed with the chyme. Bile is produced from the gall bladder, and it acts to help in the digestion and absorption of fats because of the bile salts it contains. Maltose is broken down into glucose by an enzyme called maltose, and milk sugar (lactose) and sucrose are broken down by similar enzymes. The sugars are then absorbed through the intestinal wall into the bloodstream.

Protein digestion works by using several enzymes as a team. Enzymes called trypsin and chemotrypsin break the proteins into smaller lengths, and then carboxypeptidase and aminopeptidase start removing one amino acid at a time from opposite ends of the protein molecules. This teamwork allows for faster hydrolysis of the proteins. The DNA and RNA present in food are digested in a similar team mechanism by nuclease enzymes. Very little of the fat content in a meal is digested before it reaches the small intestine. Bile salts coat droplets of fats and emulsify them so there is a large surface area for the lipase enzyme to attack. This produces glycerides, fatty acids and glycerol. All these digestive products are absorbed in the lower sections of the small intestine. These sections have a very large surface area over which the nutrients can diffuse into the blood and lymph fluids. Some sugars, e.g. fructose, diffuses across the epithelium while amino acids, glucose, vitamins and other sugars have to be pumped across the membranes. The glycerol and fatty acids recombine to form fats, and these may bind to special proteins to form lipoproteins, e.g. cholesterol. Amino acids, nucleotides and sugars travel to the liver, and from there to the heart and the rest of the body. Water in the diet is re-absorbed through the large intestine, and any undigested material is moved down the intestine to the rectum. Faeces are stored there until they are eliminated. Some beneficial bacteria live in the large intestine, including those that produce vitamin K. Most of our daily needs of this vitamin can be met by the production of these bacteria.

The nutritional benefits derived from food can be lost if there is a disorder of the stomach, liver, intestines or any of the associated enzyme-producing glands. Absorption of some vitamins and minerals is affected by disorders of the liver, pancreas or gall bladder, and also by the presence of dietary fibre or other vitamins and minerals. Copper and zinc compete to be absorbed into the body, while absorption of calcium is affected by the presence of vitamin D, stomach acids, fibre and the intake of proteins.

Interaction of medicine and nutrient absorption

Throughout the industrialized world medicines are extensively used to treat disease. Each person in Europe receives an average of five prescriptions each year. Many medicines are prescribed for more minor problems, and this may be because of pressure on the doctor rather than the necessity of the drugs for a cure to be obtained. Nearly half of all prescriptions are not used, and many of those utilized are not taken according to the doctor's instructions. Medicines affect the uptake of nutrients, vitamins and minerals into the body. Conversely, food can affect the absorption and effectiveness of many drugs. Some drugs should be taken on an empty stomach or before food so that they are rapidly digested and enter the bloodstream. Most medicines are best taken along with a meal, but this can delay absorption of the drug by two to five hours. All medicines are absorbed in the small intestine, where they compete for absorption with sugars, amino acids, nucleotides, vitamins, minerals and fats. Potassium can restrict uptake of the heart drug digoxin, while calcium, iron, zinc and magnesium form organic metal compounds with the common antibiotic tetracycline so it is not properly absorbed.

Dietary fibre can absorb a proportion of medications so that it is removed from the body instead of entering the bloodstream. Certain medicines promote the formation of oxygen-free radicals, which are discussed later (see following section, 'Dangers to our cells'). Prescribed medicines should be used carefully as some can affect the appetite and lead to nutritional problems while others, e.g. diuretic drugs, can lead to the excess elimination of some minerals, e.g. potassium and magnesium, and possible deficiency.

Dangers to our cells

Each and every one of our cells has a specific life-span, which can range from approximately 110 to 120 years for brain cells to several days for some cell types. Not all cells last to their full potential as many substances can damage them and their processes. This cell death or damage gradually builds up over time, leading to illness that may reduce our life-span. Four main processes cause damage to cells:
—oxygen-free radicals
—lipid peroxidation
—degradation of the protein molecules
—cell changes or mutations

These changes are derived from our environment and lifestyle, not our genetic inheritance.

Free radicals are chemicals that have one or more unpaired electrons in their outer shell. They are therefore highly reactive. Free radicals are produced naturally in humans as they are vital for normal functioning of the body, but they can also be generated by certain drugs and by a process called reperfusion injury. Free radicals in humans are mainly oxygen-free radicals, which can form compounds that damage our health. The most common oxygen-free radicals are superoxide (O_2-), hydrogen peroxide (H_2O_2), hydroxyl radical ($OH-$) and singlet oxygen. When produced, they exist for a very short time, possibly only a fraction of a second. Despite their short duration, they still attack the cell structure and cause damage. They attack the fatty acids that make up the membranes of all cells and oxidize them. This makes the fats rancid and damages the membrane structure of the cell. The lipids in the membrane are changed into lipid peroxides, which allow the formation of new free radicals. This chain reaction, where free radicals are regenerated, eventually leads to the destruction of the cell. Lipid peroxides can be released into the bloodstream, e.g. oxidized LDL-cholesterol, which causes irritation of the artery walls and increases the risk of arteriosclerosis. These chemicals also inhibit the formation of PGI2, prostacyclin, a prostaglandin that stops blood clots forming in the blood vessels. The oxidized fats in the membrane can degrade to form harmful prostaglandins and a toxic chemical called malonaldehyde, which can cause mutations in the genetic material of cells.

Free radicals can damage the connective tissue. Collagen makes up 30 per cent of our body's protein, and it is found in the muscles, sinews, bones and cartilage, compared to elastin, which is a connective tissue found in the skin, the artery walls and the walls of the air sacs in the lungs. Free radicals cause cross-linkages between the collagen and elastin fibres, so reducing their ability to move, stretch and bend. This means the skin and other connective tissues go hard and stiff and age quickly. Cross-linkages can lead to modifications of the blood vessels and arteriosclerosis. Action of the free radicals may cause increased levels of ageing pigments, e.g. melamine, ceroid and lipofuscin, to develop in the nerves, internal organs, the skin and the grey matter of the brain. Free radicals may also oxidize and destroy large carbohydrate molecules, which would normally be used to form mucous. Mucous acts as a joint lubricant, so free radicals can lead to joint problems.

People who are overweight have higher levels of oxidized fats in their bodies and so a greater risk of heart infarction and arteriosclerosis. Animal experiments in which the calorific intake of the animals was restricted showed an increased life-span. When this was combined with the addition of antioxidants to their diet it prevented the formation of cancer. This is because antioxidants work to protect our bodies against free radicals, lipid peroxidation, harmful chemicals, and even cancer. Natural antioxidants in our diet include vitamins A, C and E, beta-carotene, zinc and selenium. Many chronic and long-term illnesses are thought to be associated with the destructive actions of free radicals. During a heart attack the blood flow in the coronary arteries is constricted, and the area is deprived of oxygen. When normal blood flow resumes, large quantities of oxygen-free radicals are formed, and these attack the damaged cells of the heart. They oxidize some of the cellular lipids and increase the chances of another heart attack or of cardiac arrhythmia developing. Cataracts would appear to develop because of free radicals. There are normally large quantities of natural antioxidants in the eye as the retinal cells are vulnerable to attack by free radicals. A malfunction in the oxygen metabolism, caused by light and free radicals, is commonly believed to cause cataracts. Eye problems can develop in babies kept in incubators. If the oxygen dose is not monitored closely, then oxygen radicals can damage the eye. The eyesight can be protected, thankfully, by supplements of vitamin E, which removes the free radicals.

The brain is also at risk from free radicals, as it contains a lot of unsaturated fatty acids, e.g. lecithin. If these lipids are oxidized, increased amounts of lipofuscin appear in the brain. Lipofuscin is one of the ageing pigments, which, when present in large quantities, speeds up the ageing process so the person becomes prematurely senile. In Alzheimer's disease, a specific group of brain cells develops a dark brown coloration as a result of oxidized fat in the cell structure. The production of free radicals is promoted by exposure to sunlight, environmental pollutants, ozone, X-rays, and cigarette smoke. A large range of medicines can also lead to more free radicals being formed. These include antibiotics, paracetamol, anti-epileptic medicines, cytotoxic drugs, theophyllin (for asthma), the antibiotic nitrofurantoin, which is used to treat urinary tract infections, and some psychopharmaceutical drugs. The list of diseases that are believed to be caused or exacerbated by free radicals increases all the time as the results of more clinical studies are obtained. Some examples are:

alcoholic liver/heart conditions	arthritis
auto-immune diseases	arteriosclerosis
circulation disturbances	cancer
coronary heart disease	cataract
emphysema of the lung	diabetes
inflammatory reactions	liver cirrhosis
multiple sclerosis (MS)	malaria
neuronal lipofuscinosis	porphyria
premature ageing	Parkinson's disease
retinal diseases	senile dementia
rheumatoid diseases	side effects of medicines

Fortunately, we have a range of natural antioxidants that can defend our cells from free radicals and their harmful effects.

The antioxidant system

In the human body, vitamins, minerals, amino acids and specific enzymes work in cooperation to form the antioxidant system. These chemicals react with and neutralize free radicals, and they break the circle whereby free radicals degrade fatty acids and proteins, leading to the production of more free radicals and eventually causing the death of the cells. Effective antioxidants are selenium, zinc, manganese, copper, ubiquinone (co-enzyme Q10), vitamins A, C, E, B_1 (thiamine), B_3 (niacin), B_6 (pyroxidine) and possibly rutin, one of the group of bioflavonoids. Folic acid (vitamin B_9) and chemicals found in garlic and onions also have antioxidant qualities. Some amino acids, beta-carotene and some medicines also work as antioxidants. We obtain antioxidants from various sources, including tinned and processed foodstuffs. Antioxidants are added to food to prevent them from going rancid and to increase their shelf life, and this process has increased the average amount of antioxidants in our diets and reduced the incidence of diseases such as cancer or heart disease. Unfortunately, most people do not receive a high enough level of antioxidants in their normal diet to protect their health fully. Supplements of a combination of antioxidants can help protect all our cells from cancer, premature ageing and heavy metals, and aid the immune system.

The most important cells are those of the brain. Twenty per cent of the brain by weight is made up of polyunsaturated fatty acids, which are especially vulnerable to turning rancid. Recent evidence has shown that the ageing process in the brain is caused by these fatty acids being oxidized by free radicals. Most of the nervous system is also at risk, as nerve endings and the sheath around the nerves are composed of fatty material. The rancid fat is called lipofuscin, melamine and ceroid, or age pigments. If the nerve endings are oxidized, the senses of touch, smell, hearing, sight and taste can be affected. So nature has seen to it that the most vital cells in our brain are protected by large quantities of antioxidants. The spinal fluid that bathes the brain has a vitamin C content ten times that of the blood. In brain cells, vitamin C levels are 100 times that of the blood. The lens of the eye is also protected by high levels of vitamin C. So vitamin C is stored in areas where its antioxidant effects are most needed. Results from a series of controlled clinical studies showed that selenium, vitamin E, zinc and other antioxidants were effective in delaying the onset of degenerative diseases and stopping premature ageing.

Antioxidants such as zinc, vitamin E and selenium act against toxic heavy metals like cadmium, lead, mercury and aluminium. They reduce the level of damage done to the tissues by these elements. Selenium reacts with mercury so it cannot harm our cells. Selenium and vitamin E can reduce the unpleasant side effects of cytotoxic drugs, which are used during chemotherapy, for example. Most minerals, vitamins, amino acids and essential fatty acids all play a very important role in the immune system.

The immune system

The immune system is made up of four major parts:
(a) cell-mediated immune response;

235

(b) humoral (antibody-mediated) immune response;
(c) white blood cells;
(d) complement system.

The first part of our defence against pathogens is the skin, mucous membranes and their secretions. If intact, this stops most bacteria and viruses from entering the body. If entry does occur, then the inflammatory response with its phagocytic white blood cells and antimicrobial proteins kick-starts. These antimicrobial proteins are the complement system and interferons. Complement is a group of over 20 proteins that can cause lysis of invading microbes as well as acting as chemical messengers for the white blood cells. Interferons are produced by a pathogen-infected cell and alert the neighbouring cells so they cannot become infected. It reduces the spread of infection and can also activate the phagocytes and improve their function. The inflammatory response produces increased heat and blood flow to the affected area with swelling. Chemical signals such as histamine or prostaglandins are released, and they have several actions. Phagocytes such as neutrophils and macrophages arrive at the injury, and they kill any pathogens by ingesting them and destroying them with enzymes. They also ingest debris of the cells that were damaged. Inflammatory reactions can be localized or found throughout the system. In some cases, molecules called pyrogens are released from white blood cells, and these trigger a fever to try and help the body fight the pathogen. These immune responses are nonspecific, and they occur in response to bacteria, viruses or physical injury in exactly the same manner.

The white blood cells are heavily involved in the specific immune response. There are five major types of white cells. Monocytes and neutrophils are phagocytic cells involved in the inflammatory response. Monocytes can develop into macrophages, which have an important role in cellular immunity. Basophils and eosinophils also work in the inflammatory reaction, while lymphocytes are the cells that produce antibodies or attack and kill pathogens.

The specific immune responses are derived from the humoral (antibody-mediated) or the cell-mediated response systems. Both B- and T-cells develop from stem cells in the bone marrow. When pathogens enter the body, they are termed 'antigen' (antibody-generating). Antigens include viruses, bacteria, protozoans, fungi and parasitic worms. When an antigen is encountered in the body, it generally meets one of the white blood cells, or leucocytes. The antigen may be taken up by a macrophage, which then changes into an antigen-presenting cell to warn other sections of the immune system of the invader.

A helper T-cell is triggered by this antigen-presenting cell, and it acts in two ways. It stimulates the humoral immune response to produce B-lymphocytes, which are made in the bone marrow. The B-cells produce two cell types—plasma cells and memory B-cells—both of which are specific to the original antigen. The plasma cells go on to make antibodies, which are specific to the pathogen, and they are released into the blood and lymph fluid to locate and bind to their specific antigenic pathogen. The memory B-cells survive in the body fluids for long periods and are reactivated, if and when they encounter the original antigen again, to provide a rapid response by producing antibodies and more memory cells. The memory cells allow a faster and stronger immune response to repeated exposure to an antigen, and this mechanism can confer lifelong immunity from certain pathogens, e.g. measles, chickenpox.

The activated helper T-cell also stimulates the cell-mediated immune response by activating cytotoxic T-cells. They are the only cell-killing T-cells, and they locate, bind to and then lyse infected cells. This prevents further reproduction of the pathogen and exposes the pathogen to the B-cell antibody response, hence increasing its success. Like B-cells, T-cells also produce memory T-cells to provide a faster immune reaction upon further contact with the specific antigen. Both B-cells and cytotoxic T-cells can be stimulated by free antigens in the blood or lymph fluid without the action of a helper T-cell.

The T-lymphocytes that make up the cell-mediated response move from their source in the bone marrow to the thymus gland in the upper chest to develop fully. Here they mature and differentiate into two classes; the regulator T-cells and the effector T-cells. Regulator T-cells are the helper T-cells and suppressor T-cells that control the activities of both T- and B-lymphocytes. The effector T-cells are the killer T-cells and delayed hypersensitivity T-cells. The killer T-cell is the only cell that kills the pathogen and infected cells. These B-cells remain and mature in the bone marrow and have the two classes; antibody-producing cells and memory cells. Speculation continues as to whether there is a set of regulatory B-cells that has not yet been found.

Without a healthy and effective immune system, the body would be considerably weakened and far more affected by everyday viruses or bacterial infections. It has long been known that vitamins and some trace elements are essential to the production of some immune cells, antibodies or chemical signals in the body, and continued medical research confirms this. Our daily requirement of vitamins may be small, but they have a considerable impact on the normal functioning of our immune system and energy metabolism.

Allergy and auto-immune diseases

Problems can arise with the immune system where it turns against itself. This leads to a series of auto-immune diseases, such as rheumatoid arthritis, Grave's disease or systemic lupus erythematosus (SLE). These problems can be especially difficult to treat or control.

Counting Calories

Allergies occur because the body's defences are hypersensitive to some allergens in our environment. The inflammatory response releases histamines and other inflammatory agents into the bloodstream, and the person may start sneezing with a runny nose and even have breathing difficulties. Both the cell and antibody-mediated immune response overreact to antigens, producing an allergic reaction. Most allergens are things like pollen, dust (or more specifically the house dust mite), cats, dogs or horses. Food allergy also occurs and has a range of severity. The most severe form of allergic reaction is anaphylactic shock, when a person can have breathing difficulties, swelling of the throat, a drop in blood pressure and loss of consciousness. Here, death can occur within minutes unless adrenaline is administered to counteract the allergic response. This type of allergic reaction is fortunately fairly rare but can be caused by a bee or wasp sting or by eating nuts, especially peanuts, or shellfish.

At the other end of the scale, some people can be sensitive to some foods, and this may cause problems such as migraines, respiratory difficulties, tension, depression, joints and muscle aches, and headaches. Other conditions, such as hay fever symptoms, irritability, cramps, stomach upsets and indigestion, may also result from food intolerance. The most common type of food sensitivity is to dairy products or wheat. It may be difficult to pinpoint any specific food that triggers a reaction, but it may be worthwhile eliminating a suspect food from your diet for a time and seeing if the symptoms alleviate.

Some nutritional doctors believe that allergies can be treated and eased by supplementation with certain vitamins, minerals and essential fatty acids. Adults with an adverse reaction to pollen and dogs have had their symptoms removed by taking selenium and calcium tablets each day. Children allergic to horses and milk and suffering from asthma have been 'cured' of these problems by treatment with zinc, selenium and gamma-linolenic acid. Asthma patients treated in this manner have noticed a reduction in respiratory difficulties and in mucous formation in the lungs. In some cases, people have no longer required their normal medical treatment of steroid pills and inhalers. It must be noted that each case of allergy or asthma is treated individually, and benefits derived from nutritional supplements can vary. In asthma, inflammation of the bronchi plays a large part in the condition, and free radicals are known to be involved in inflammatory responses. Asthma and allergies are activated by prostaglandins and the immune system. People with allergies have higher levels of the antibody immunoglobulin E (IgE) in their bodies, which is under the control of the B-cells. The B-cells are also controlled by the T-cells, and it is the T-cells that weaken faster as we grow older. Thus, reduced activity of the T-cells, particularly a group called the suppressor T-cells, which normally tells an immune response to stop, is linked to auto-immune diseases and allergies, asthma and arthritis. So supplements to boost the functioning of the T-cells would be beneficial. Zinc can stimulate the hormone thymulin and interleukin-2, which both activate T-cells. Essential fatty acids such as gamma-linolenic acid, eicosapentanoic acid (EPA) and docosahexanoic acid (DHA) help regulate the protaglandin and leukotriene metabolisms and temper the inflammatory response. Antioxidants can be taken to fight the free radicals produced in the inflammatory response.

The role of vitamins, minerals and essential fatty acids in the immune system

Supplements of iron, selenium, zinc, copper, magnesium, vitamins A, C, D, E and B_6 along with gamma-linolenic acid, EPA and DHA can help to strengthen the immune system and prevent recurrent viral infections. The dosage needed is much greater than that found in our normal diets, but the benefits of fewer infections are well worth it. Children from six months to four years old were also given a range of supplements, and they had a reduced incidence of common infectious diseases such as ear infections, colds and sinusitis.

Vitamins and minerals are required for the formation and functioning of many immune cells. Deficiencies of vitamin A, B_1 (thiamin), B_3 (niacin) or C result in specific disease conditions, which can be resolved by sufficient intake of that vitamin. Viral and bacterial infections reduce the levels of vitamin A, B_6 and C in the body, and higher levels of vitamin B_2 (riboflavin) are eliminated during a fever. All the B vitamins and vitamin C are essential to the normal functioning of white blood cells in an inflammatory response. The defence mechanisms of the macrophages and the T- and B-lymphocytes require vitamins A, B_1, B_2, B_9 (folic acid), B_{12} and E to function well. Many vitamins, including A, B_6, B_9 and B_{12}, take part in making proteins and DNA, so lack of any of them can result in reduced resistance to disease. Vitamin B_6 (pyridoxine) encourages production of nucleic acids in cells that are crucial for growth and the production of antibodies. The thymus gland, where the T-lymphocytes are matured, also depends on vitamin B_6. Pyroxidine deficiency leads to fewer T- and B-lymphocytes in the blood and fewer antibodies produced. Lack of B_6 means neutrophil white blood cells are less able to ingest and destroy bacteria. Infants born to mothers with inadequate pyroxidine levels have a smaller spleen and thymus than normal children, so newborn children with deficiencies in vitamins may have a weakened cellular immunity. Up to a third of elderly people may lack enough vitamin B_6, and this can reduce their resistance to ageing and illness, and may even impair their mental functions. Lowered levels of antibody production may occur because of inadequate supplies of vitamin A, B_6, B_5 (pantothenic acid), B_9 and biotin.

239

Vitamins A, C and E help to protect the mucous membranes and the skin. Too little vitamin A can mean a smaller thymus and spleen, hence fewer white blood cells being produced. Children born with insufficient vitamin A are far more at risk from infectious diseases, and supplements given to children in Indonesia and Africa resulted in lowered child mortality. Care should be taken, as too much vitamin A is toxic and has the effect of weakening the immune system. Vitamin C's role is to make sure the skin is strong and to maintain the correct working of the neutrophils. It may be worthwhile increasing our intake of vitamin C during colds or influenza, for example, as the level of the vitamin in the macrophages falls, so impairing their ability to fight the pathogen. Lack of vitamin E weakens antibody formation, the activity of the lymphocytes, and causes changes in the delayed hypersensitivity reaction.

Certain minerals also have their part to play in the immune system. The metabolism of zinc changes when our bodies are fighting infection. The zinc is used to produce a protein that helps to protect our cells, but if the infection continues for a period of time we may become deficient in the mineral. A contributory factor is that the loss of zinc via the urine and excreta increases during an infection, and the uptake via the diet may be less because of lack of appetite. Since zinc is involved with the functioning of nearly 200 enzymes, lack of zinc can lead to all sorts of problems, including less energy being produced in the cells and no formation of nucleic acids. Zinc helps cells divide, so is vital to the proliferation and maturation of lymphocytes. Zinc is particularly important for the helper T-cells and the killer cells of the inflammatory response. Insufficient zinc affects the thymus in a similar manner to lack of vitamin A, with reduced hormone production but increased antibody formation.

Iron is necessary for the functioning of the lymph tissues and also for the correct activity of the neutrophils. Lack of iron can disrupt the immune system, damaging the cellular immunity, and occasionally the antibody levels may drop as well. Disruption to the immune system from lack of iron can occur when our intake is reduced by only 10 per cent. This may be because of an accompanying deficiency in vitamin B_9, folic acid. Iron forms part of enzyme proteins like transferrin and lactoferrin. These proteins scavenge all the available iron, so none is left for bacteria and they cannot grow. People suffering from long-term infections or inflammation are often anaemic and lacking iron. When given supplements, the anaemia is still present as the iron is taken into the blood serum and the tissues, not the red blood cells. When this occurs, the enzyme proteins are saturated with iron, and any pathogens can grow without restriction on the available iron. Thus, it actually increases the risk of developing new infections. In the case of some rheumatoid arthritis patients, they may have too much iron but their levels of haemoglobin in the blood are low. Here, the iron is held in the blood serum and tissues, and the number of red blood cells is dangerously low. This shows that iron supplementation may not always help fight disease.

During infections, the levels of copper (in the form of the protein ceruloplasmin) in the blood increase. This is believed to play a part in the body's defence mechanism but is not yet fully understood. Magnesium and calcium are both needed so that the metabolism of cell membranes can function normally. Lack of magnesium weakens formation of antibodies and leads to reduced size of the thymus gland. During infection, the levels of magnesium in the blood fall, and the body loses a lot of the calcium and magnesium that are released from the cells. Magnesium supplements would seem to be critical where a large amount of the mineral is lost because of serious burns or complications after an operation. The mineral helps the formation of complement proteins and acts to prevent allergies and common infections.

Lack of selenium reduces the cellular immune system, particularly if the person is deficient in vitamin E. Selenium allows the neutrophils to destroy antigens and boosts the activity of the T-lymphocytes. Inadequate selenium levels lead to increased lipid peroxidation in cell membranes, and deficiency of selenium and vitamin E at the same time increases the risk of developing cancer.

Vitamins and cancer

Cancer is a disease of disordered cell growth. Certain cells start uncontrolled growth to form a tumour that may invade surrounding tissues and spread by a process called metastasis to form secondary tumours in other parts of the body. Cancer develops in phases, starting with initiation, then promotion and progression to form a malignant tumour. Initiation occurs when DNA molecules inside a cell are attacked by a carcinogen. This substance can cause irreversible damage to DNA in a very short time. Some cancers develop without any damage being done to the DNA. The change in DNA that results is called a mutation. Carcinogens may be natural or synthetic in origin, and we are exposed to them in the air, sunlight, air pollution, our diet and our lifestyle. This damage to our DNA happens all the time, and in most of us our internal repair system prevents any problem developing and replaces the damaged DNA. If this does not occur, the disease can progress. This disease-causing initiation can occur often as a result of many tiny mutations that may occur day after day.

The next stage is the promotion phase. Here the cell with the mutation undergoes a number of chain reactions, which produce a cancer cell. The body loses control of the cell, which starts to divide uncontrollably. The tumour formed is a mass of genetically identical

241

cells. Substances that promote cell division and proliferation can act as promoters. These include excessive oestrogen, arsenic, epoxides, excessive exposure to sunlight and lack of vitamin A. This promotion stage is called 'precancerous' by doctors. Progression or clonal evolution follows the promotion stage. Here the cell population in the tumour produces clones of cells, which are slightly different genetically from the original tumour and from each other. These cells have a high division rate; they move into other tissues and send out metastases (daughter tumours) to other areas of the body. When examined under a microscope, the cells look different and disorganized. Doctors call this dysplasia and say they are 'premalignant' as they have not infiltrated other tissues. When this occurs, they are considered malignant and cancerous. The promotion and progression phases are difficult, if not impossible, to separate as the process is a continuum that results in a fully developed cancer.

Cancer exists in many different forms, which are classified according to the cells that gave rise to them. The most common types are carcinomas of the skin, glands and the membranes lining the respiratory, urinary and gastrointestinal systems. Sarcomas develop from connective tissues, cartilage, muscles and membranes covering muscles and fat, and are less common. Lymphoma is cancer of the lymph nodes while leukaemia is a disease of the white blood cells. The treatment of each type is different as are the causes and specific progression of the disease. In the UK, the commonest cancers are of the lungs, the breasts and the skin. Around 90 per cent of all lung cancers are caused by smoking, and there is increasing evidence that passive smoking can contribute to developing the disease. Lung cancer is also difficult to cure, and only 10 per cent of patients survive for longer than 10 years. Skin cancer is easier to treat and has a higher success rate if the disease is caught early enough. There are 25,000 new cases a year, and this number is increasing as more people take sunshine holidays and are exposed to more ultraviolet light. There is the possibility that the reduced levels of ozone in the upper atmosphere is letting more ultraviolet light through to the ground, and this may result in more cancers developing.

Breast cancer is the most common cancer in Britain, killing 15,000 women a year. Routine examination is recommended to check for lumps, and a breast screening programme for women aged between 50 and 64 is currently under way. Breast cancer may be prevented by taking anti-oestrogen drugs such as tamoxifen, by breast-feeding, by a low fat diet, and some doctors believe that nipple stimulation encourages production of a hormone called oxytocin, which is normally produced during breast-feeding and may reduce the risks of developing breast cancer. Five to ten per cent of breast cancers are thought to be linked to genetics. Two genes that are linked to breast cancer development have been found, BRCA 1 and BRCA 2, and work is continuing to find the range of possible mutations and to develop a screening programme for these genes.

Although we are exposed to carcinogens in our diet, many dietary components can also help to protect us against cancer. For example, fibre absorbs carcinogens and fat in our diet, and takes them out of our body. A diet that is high in fibre also reduces the length of time for which the digested food is present in the large intestine, so reducing the amount of time that the colon and rectum are exposed to harmful substances. This is proven to reduce the incidence of colon and rectal cancers. Evidence shows that up to 40 per cent of all cancers may be caused by nutritional factors. This is partly because of the carcinogens in food but also because of insufficient intake of protective vitamins and minerals. Recent studies have proposed that deficiencies of beta-carotene, vitamins A, C and E and selenium could increase the risks of developing cancer. Many large-scale clinical studies are under way in both hemispheres to determine the effects of these and other micronu-trients that may prevent cancer. Several nutritional doctors recommend supplements of $100\mu g$ of selenium (in the form of L-seleno-methio-nine) 30mg ubiquinone, 200–300mg of vitamin C, 200mg of vitamin E and 16,000–20,000 IU of beta-carotene per day. This may seem exces-sive but would have considerable benefits against not only cancer but also against heart disease and infectious diseases.

Many of these vitamins and minerals are also used in conjunction with chemotherapy and radiotherapy. Both these means of treating cancer can cause damage to our cells. Chemotherapy with cytotoxic drugs can kill cells other than the cancer cells and also triggers produc-tion of more free radicals in the body. Radiotherapy can kill the cancer cells but also may damage the genetic material in normal, healthy cells. These two treatments lower the levels of beta-carotene and vitamin E in the blood, so supplementation is required. There is some evidence to back the idea that beta-carotene, canthaxanthine (a provitamin of vitamin A), selenium, gamma-linolenic acid and fish oils may inhibit the proliferation of cancer cells and may also prevent or limit the devel-opment of metastases. Supplementation boosts the general condition of a person with cancer and can help the patient deal with the experi-ence of chemotherapy or radiotherapy. Some doctors believe that sup-plements of the antioxidants, vitamin A, C, E, B_1, B_2, B_3, B_6 and manga-nese and magnesium, can help a patient deal with difficult treatments. Fish oils containing EPA and DHA, gamma-linolenic acid, selenium and some amino acids may be good in helping to fight cancer.

Healthy people can tolerate repeated initiations by carcinogens as the immune system and the antioxidant defence system can disable the harmful substances and repair the damaged cellular DNA.

Counting Calories

Vitamins and heart disease

Heart diseases are the single largest killer in the UK and throughout the industrialized world. There are various forms of heart disease, the main examples being coronary thrombosis, cardiac arrhythmia, hypertension and chronic diseases of the heart valves. It may also be associated with diseases of the coronary arteries, the commonest of which is coronary arteriosclerosis. This is a progressive disease that may start developing before puberty. The arteries become narrowed by deposits of fat and oxidized fats that build up on the artery walls. These plaques harden and narrow the blood vessel, reducing the blood flow through it. The oxidized fats stop an enzyme called prostacyclin synthetase from working. The enzyme produces prostacyclin (PG12), which is normally found in the walls of the artery, and when levels of PG12 fall blood starts to clot in that area. Red blood cells in the clot rupture and release iron and copper, which stimulate oxidation and eventually lead to the formation of a blood clot. This clot can detach itself and move through the circulatory system, and it may become lodged in a blood capillary in the brain, heart or lungs. In arteriosclerosis, restricted blood flow through coronary arteries can lead to oxygen deficiency in the heart, which is known as angina pectoris. Symptoms of angina include breathlessness, dizziness and sweating with a dull pain or tightness in the chest. When the blood flow returns to normal, reperfusion of blood in the tissues occurs, and this can produce toxic-free radicals in the cells. These radicals can increase the levels of oxidized fats in the plaque. Many antioxidants in our diets can protect against these effects of free radicals and reduce the damage done to heart cells.

Antioxidants can also prevent heart failure, if given within three hours of a heart attack. So, if we improve our diet by reducing our intake of all fats, particularly saturated fats, and increase the levels of antioxidants in our bodies, then we can prevent or lessen the formation of plaques in our arteries and hence prevent blood clots and further damage. Vitamins A, C, E, B_6, along with beta-carotene, ubiquinone, selenium and zinc, all work to limit the action of oxygen radicals in the tissues of the heart and arteries. Ubiquinone (also called co-enzyme Q10) is very important in protecting the cardiac cells and is commonly prescribed to heart patients in Japan.

Many large studies have been carried out to monitor antioxidant levels in blood serum and to work out if there is a link between the antioxidant level in blood and the risk of coronary heart disease. It seems that the lower the level of antioxidant in blood, the higher the risk of death from myocardial infarction. Myocardial infarction is another term for ischaemic heart disease, or coronary heart disease. This disease results from blockage or narrowing of one of the coronary arteries, which reduces the blood supply to the heart, leading to oxygen deficiency and death of areas of heart tissue (myocardium). The heart can tolerate lack of oxygen and reperfusion of blood much better if it contains enough antioxidants. Cardiac arrhythmia may be caused by low levels of both potassium and magnesium in the blood. Tests of blood serum for these minerals do not reflect their true values, as most of the body's potassium and magnesium is found inside the cells. In some cases supplements of magnesium can help to reduce the severity of cardiac arrhythmia. Arrhythmia may also be eased by supplements of selenium, vitamins E and B_6.

Fish oils containing eicosapentaenoic acid (EPA) and docosahexanoic acid (DHA) are believed to help in cases of heart disease. These oils are rich in omega-3 fatty acids, which decrease the tendency of blood platelets to clot in the blood vessels. They seem to reduce the levels of cholesterol in the blood and also lower the levels of fat or triglycerides in the blood. Fish oils are found in fatty fish such as herring, mackerel, tuna and salmon. They generally help prevent arteriosclerosis developing and reduce the chances of blood clots forming, which may block blood vessels. People with a diet rich in fatty fish (and so fish oils) have a reduced incidence of heart disease with far less mortality.

Vitamins

vitamin A

This is a fat-soluble vitamin that occurs naturally in animal products.
It is actually a group of compounds including retinol, retinal, carotene
and carotenoids. Retinol is the main active form of vitamin A, and it
is proposed to have a hormonal function. The chemical structure of
retinol was determined by Paul Karrer in 1931, and both natural and
synthetic forms of vitamin A have been available for many years. The
carotenes are precursors to vitamin A, and when ingested they are
transformed into vitamin A in the liver. They are safer as they are nontoxic to humans and there is no risk of poisoning.

The active form of vitamin A is the aldehyde retinal, which is vital for
the proper formation of rhodopsin, the light-sensitive pigment in vertebrate rod cells in the eye. The pigment is made up of retinal attached to
the protein opsin. When light enters the eye and hits a rod cell, it stimulates a set of reactions in which rhodopsin separates back into its two
components, and this triggers nervous activity in the rod cell and sends
an image to the brain. The rhodopsin pigment reforms in darkness.
This is why vitamin A is critical for good eyesight and why it prevents
night blindness. In cases of vitamin A deficiency, various deleterious effects can occur. The epithelial tissues can atrophy, leading to conditions
called keratomalacia and xerophthalmia. Keratomalacia is a condition
in which the cornea in the eye is dry and ulcerated. This shows as night
blindness, abnormal sensitivity to light, painful conjunctiva and red and
swollen eyelids. It can eventually lead to blindness. Xerophthalmia is
a similar condition in which the cornea and conjunctiva are dry and
lustreless. Deficiency of vitamin A also leads to night blindness, defec-
tive development of the teeth, stunted growth, various skin eruptions,
problems of the mucous membranes and reduced defence against
infections. A lack of vitamin A in children in developing countries can
cause ulceration of the eye, blindness and death.

Vitamin A is found in many foods, including butter, egg yolk, animal
fats, liver, green vegetables, kidney, yellow/red fruits and yellow/orange
vegetables. In the average diet, three-quarters of our vitamin A comes
from retinol itself, while the rest comes from beta-carotene. Excess vitamin A is stored in the liver, and the vitamin has a half-life of between
200 and 300 days in the liver, so the vitamin A balance is only disturbed

246

if intake is too low over a period of months. An estimated one million IU of stored vitamin A is found in each person, 90 per cent of that in the liver, 1.5 per cent in the blood and the rest contained in other tissues. The capacity for vitamin storage is reduced in cases of liver disease.

There is a possibility that vitamin A can be stored in such large quantities that it becomes toxic. Cases are recorded where vitamin poisoning has occurred with vitamins A and D, and this normally occurs with very high doses over long periods of time. Acute vitamin A poisoning was first seen more than 100 years ago in polar explorers, who ate polar bear liver and seal meat, which is very rich in vitamin A (> 10,000 IU per gram). They suffered from dizziness, nausea, headaches and vomiting, which are classic signs of acute vitamin A poisoning. Early symptoms of excess vitamin A are dry skin and itching. Doses of approximately 25,000 IU per day should be acceptable even over a long time period. There is a risk of vitamin A overdosing in pregnancy with a risk of foetal damage, but that has been with doses in excess of 20,000 IU per day. Several doctors state that it is perfectly safe, even during pregnancy, to take daily supplements of up to 8000 IU of vitamin A.

Recent research has indicated several new areas where vitamin A or beta-carotene are important in the body. Vitamin A and the carotenoid group have become an effective treatment for a number of skin diseases, including photosensitivity, where exposure to sunlight or ultraviolet light can cause oedema, acute burns, urticaria and skin lesions. Beta-carotene is an antioxidant that can stop excess oxidation of fats or lipids in cells. This appears to work via the cell's genetic material, either RNA or DNA, although the actual mechanism is not known. Beta-carotene also has a special affinity to an oxygen-free radical called singlet oxygen. This is a compound with an extra electron or proton that is unstable and readily reacts with other molecules in the body. Beta-carotene appears to react with the radical and removes it from the system. Beta-carotene can protect the skin from excessive sunlight, and this may result in a yellowing of the skin, which is not a result of overdosing on beta-carotene.

Prophylactic treatment with vitamin A and beta-carotene

Antioxidant vitamins and minerals found naturally in our diet can protect us against the harmful effects of free radicals, lipid peroxidation and even help prevent cancer. This may seem like an extreme statement, but it is now believed that most chronic and common diseases are caused by deleterious mutations in our DNA, most of which are caused by free radicals. So, if we take enough antioxidants into our bodies, we can support our immune system and perhaps prevent the occurrence of many diseases.

Low levels of vitamin A and beta-carotene in the blood are thought to be a risk factor in cancer, and so higher doses of these two chemicals are thought to have a prophylactic effect on cancers. This beneficial effect is increased when vitamin A is combined with vitamin E and the mineral selenium, which are also antioxidants. Vitamin A has been found to reinforce the immune system and increase survival rates of children in the Third World. Many epidemiological studies have found that a low blood serum level of beta-carotene would indicate a future risk of cancer. Beta-carotene levels in the blood appear to be reduced by smoking, which is also a risk in terms of lung cancer. A major study is currently under way of 52,000 people in Finland and the United States on the effects of diet supplementation with beta-carotene on disease levels.

Disease treatment

In underdeveloped countries around 50 million children have a deficiency of vitamin A. The World Health Organization and UNICEF are running large-scale projects in Africa and southeast Asia to try to overcome this. Mothers are given 200,000 IU and children get around 100,000 IU weekly, and so far the level of xerophthalmia and blindness has fallen by more than 80 per cent, and child mortality has fallen by 35 per cent. These periodic huge doses of vitamin A are not ideal, but it is effective in these difficult areas. Vitamin A helps in the renewal of skin cells and in replacement of the collagen (proteins in the connective tissues), so it has been given to help treat certain skin diseases. Acne can be helped with a daily intake of 100,000–200,000 IU over a period of weeks or months. The dosage is normally reduced after a few weeks. A vitamin A derivative called tretinon is used as a lotion, gel or cream and is often prescribed by doctors to treat acne with lesions, pustules and blackheads. Its use must be carefully monitored as the lotion can cause irritation of the eyes, nose and mouth, and there can be an adverse reaction to excess ultraviolet or sunlight exposure. It is a common and highly effective treatment in most cases.

Other skin diseases that can benefit from vitamin A treatment include psoriasis, where patients were given very high doses of up to 300,000 IU per day. This involved a risk of toxicity so a new derivative of vitamin A, called isotretinoid, has been used for treating psoriasis. These isotretinoid chemicals are actually thirty times more concentrated than vitamin A and are of particular risk if pregnant. The preparations are marketed as Retin-A lotion and as Roaccutane capsules, but they are available only on prescription. This new vitamin A product has also been used in some forms of cancer, e.g. T-cell leukaemia.

Vitamin A and beta-carotene are also given to cancer patients undergoing cytotoxic chemotherapy or radiotherapy. The treatment produces free radicals in the body, which are supposed to attack cancer cells, but they also damage normal tissue and reduce the level of natural antioxidant chemicals in the blood. Work carried out in Italy has shown that supplementation of beta-carotene with a vitamin A derivative called canthaxanthine has anti-cancer properties that may stop the formation of daughter tumours. Clinical studies are currently proceeding to examine these results more closely.

The recommended dietary allowances for vitamin A are 5000 IU in Europe and the USA, which equals about 1mg. The values of RDA are based on American figures, which were first calculated in 1943 and are updated every five years. They apply only to the healthy population and exclude babies, pregnant and nursing mothers, people with chronic or infectious diseases, people on permanent medication, people with metabolic disorders, smokers and people aged over 50. The RDAs are calculated with an inbuilt safety margin and are only the vitamin levels required to prevent well-known deficiency symptoms. Today, there is much more awareness of the preventative nature of vitamins and minerals, and doses well above RDA levels are common in preventing disease and boosting the immune system.

Beta-carotene itself can be considered an essential vitamin. It is a powerful antioxidant and a cancer prophylactic, with recommended blood serum levels set at 400 nano moles per litre. It can be given for hypersensitivity to light and photo-allergy, which can occur in the chronic disease known as systemic lupus erythematosus (SLE). Beta-carotene can also help absorb the free radicals produced by reperfusion in humans. Reperfusion is another name for the oxidation damage that occurs in cells that have been deprived of oxygen because of a reduced blood supply. When the blood flow returns to normal and the tissues are supplied with oxygen, some damage occurs because of the large amounts of oxygen radicals that are produced. These radicals can be neutralized by antioxidants, so reducing the level of damage caused to cells and also the impact on the cells. This type of oxidation damage is a risk in coronary heart disease, thrombosis, arteriosclerosis, brain circulatory disorders and in all types of surgery. It is a particular problem with hand or heart surgery where the circulation is stopped for a time and in transplant operations. There is a link between reperfusion injury and arrhythmia where reperfusion raises the number of oxygen radicals formed and they attack the fatty acids in the cell membranes to form toxic aldehydes and lipoxins, which can stimulate possibly fatal arrhythmia. Antioxidants including beta-carotene, selenium, etc, can inhibit the action of the oxygen radicals and stop any damage occurring in the heart cells.

vitamin B₁

thiamin, thiamine, aneurine

Vitamin B$_1$ is part of the vitamin B complex, and is water-soluble and hence easily lost during food preparation. Thiamin cannot be stored in the body in large quantities as there are only small reserve areas in the liver, heart and brain, and any excess is removed in the urine. The chemical structure of thiamin was discovered in 1936 by Robert Williams, and its main action in the body is in the formation of the enzyme thiamin pyrophosphate. This enzyme is required for the decarboxylation of certain acids in the Krebs cycle and is involved in the conversion of alanine to acetyl co-enzyme A, which is essential to the process. Thiamin also promotes normal metabolism, appetite, digestion and growth in the body, and it is also essential for the health of the cardiovascular and nervous systems. Thiamin also improves the functioning of T-cells and is required for normal development and functioning of the brain.

Deficiency of this vitamin can have a range of effects. It is thought that about half the population in industrialized countries suffers from minor long-term vitamin B deficiency. The RDA for thiamin is 1.5mg, but various factors increase the level required, e.g. pregnant women and elderly people need more thiamin per day. Factors such as stress, operations, alcohol, medicine, tobacco and carbohydrate consumption all affect the level of vitamin B_1 needed. Some of the thiamin taken into the body is not used for its original purpose, as it is consumed by alcohol, tobacco, stimulants such as coffee, and hormonal contraceptive pills. Minor deficiency may cause anxiety, irritability and depression, but the symptoms change as the deficiency becomes more severe. Ultimately, lack of thiamine leads to a disease called beriberi in which there is nerve inflammation with muscular weakness and heart failure. Loss of weight and appetite, disordered nerve function causing paralysis and wasting of limbs can also become part of the disease, which is common in Japan and other eastern areas. The disease is easily cleared up by a supplement of thiamin. Absorption of thiamin in the body occurs through the small intestine, and uptake of the vitamin is disrupted by disturbances in nutrient absorption, anorexia nervosa, chronic poor general health with diarrhoea and vomiting, and the use of diuretic medicines. Also, alcoholics often have thiamin deficiency, which can lead to weakening of the heart muscle and possibly heart failure.

Thiamin has no particular toxic effects, even in large doses of greater than 300 times the RDA. If given as an injection, vitamin B_1 can cause toxic symptoms like shaking, nervousness, swelling, disturbance of heart rhythm and allergic reactions. This may proceed further to disturb the functioning of the heart and nerves. These problems are resolved purely by cutting down the dose or stopping thiamin supplementation totally.

Thiamin is an antioxidant in humans, along with its fellow B vitamins—pantothenic acid B_5, B_3 niacin and B_2 riboflavin—and it is said to protect the cells from the chemical acetaldehyde, which is formed in cells by the action of free radicals. Acetaldehyde can cause mutations in DNA and cause cancer. Thiamin has been used as a medicine in skin diseases, disturbances in heart function, cancer, arteriosclerosis and arthritis to remove the free radicals produced by those diseases. Thiamin can also benefit a smoker's cough, seasickness, toothache and other minor pains. The B vitamins are synergistic in effect, i.e. they reinforce each other's effects on the body, and hence thiamin is best taken as part of a vitamin B complex supplement.

The best sources of thiamin are yeast, grain husks, whole-wheat products, peas, beans, potatoes, nuts, liver, eggs and pork. Deficiency can result from poorly milled or polished rice, which has lost most of its vitamin B_1 content.

vitamin B_2
riboflavin, lactoflavin, vitamin G
Vitamin B_2 or riboflavin is a water-soluble vitamin that can be partially decomposed by heat and sunlight. It was first detected in 1879 by Blyth, and its structure was isolated in 1935 by Paul Karrer and Richard Kuhn, among others. The vitamin has a crystalline structure and is yellow-orange in colour.

Riboflavin is found in various foodstuffs, including milk, liver, eggs, cheese, fish, yoghurt, green vegetables, pulses and yeast extract. Deficiencies of this vitamin can occur in pregnant mothers, nursing women, the elderly, slimmers, vegans and the chronically ill. Lack of riboflavin can be caused by diseases such as arthritis and tuberculosis, and by the action of drugs like antibiotics, tranquillizers, contraceptive pills and sulpha products. Vitamin B_2 in the body is absorbed by the small intestine, and the process is regulated by thyroid gland hormones. Thus some antidepressants and nerve medicines can affect the thyroid and disrupt absorption of the vitamin. Riboflavin is largely stored in our red blood cells, and reserves in the human body seem to be fairly stable, with any excess being eliminated in the urine or excreta. Vitamin B_2 deficiency can result in inflammation of the tongue and lips, scaly scalp and eczema, hair loss, dizziness, insomnia, hacks in the corner of the mouth and oversensitivity to light. Some studies indicate that riboflavin deficiency is the commonest vitamin deficiency in industrialized countries, with 20 per cent of people suffering from it. Riboflavin has an important role in energy release from carbohydrates, in that it forms part of two co-enzymes called flavine adenine dinucleotide (FAD) and flavine mononucleotide (FMN). These chemicals are involved in the metabolism of all nutrients as well as being two critical components of the oxidative phosphorylation reactions of the electron transport chain. This means that the food eaten is broken down efficiently and the maximum energy is obtained from it.

Riboflavin is also involved in the production of the brain neurotransmitters serotonin, noradrenaline and acetylcholine and in histamine, which is released from tissue cells after damage. It is also connected to the synthesis of the three essential fatty acids required by humans—linoleic acid, linolenic acid and arachidonic acid. Riboflavin inhibits the production of chemicals called leukotrienes and prostaglandins. Prostaglandins are a group of unsaturated fatty acids that are found in most mammalian tissues. They have a wide range of activity on the body, including regulation of cell function and fertility. They lower blood pressure and cause contraction of smooth muscle. They are released after tissue damage as part of the inflammatory response and can cause painful muscle cramps in some people.

There is very little risk of overdosing on riboflavin as the upper limit is 3g per kilogram of body weight per day and the RDA is 1.3mg–1.7mg per day. Extremely large doses can cause numbness and itching in some cases.

vitamin B$_3$

niacin, nicotinic acid, nicotinamide, nicotinate; chemical name: pyridine-3-carboxylic acid, $C_5 H_4 N$ COOH

Unlike vitamins B$_1$ and B$_2$, niacin can be produced in the body from the essential amino acid tryptophan. This only occurs in small amounts so most of the human requirements are met in our diet. Niacin is a white, crystalline vitamin that is water-soluble and hence vulnerable to destruction by heat, strong light and low temperatures.

Vitamin B$_3$ is contained in meat, poultry, liver, kidney, eggs, nuts, fish, cheese, peas, beans, milk, dried fruit, yeast extract and some cereals, e.g. rice. It is found as two different forms—nicotinic acid and its amide, nicotinamide, both of which are active in the body. Niacin has various beneficial actions, and it is critical to food metabolism and the breakdown of glucose in the Krebs cycle. Niacin is used biosynthetically to derive the co-enzyme nicotinamide adenine dinucleotide (NAD), which is essential to a large number of oxidation reduction reactions that occur in the breakdown of glucose and fatty acids to release energy. NAD also exists as NADP, with an additional phosphate group. Niacin also plays a part in maintenance of the nervous system, normal functioning of the gastrointestinal tract, maintenance of healthy skin, and synthesis of the sex hormones. It also aids efficient blood circulation by expanding the arteries and reducing resistance to blood flow. Niacin is known to remove low-density lipoprotein cholesterol from the blood. This LDL-cholesterol is the dangerous form of cholesterol that increases the risk of hardening of the coronary arteries. This suggests that niacin may be beneficial in preventing heart disease.

Other therapeutic uses of niacin are to treat dizziness and contracted blood vessels, as well as using niacin in conjunction with other B complex vitamins to reduce fluid loss from the body associated with burns. Vitamin B_3 has been used in the United States as a substitute for sleeping pills, and it has been utilized as a tranquillizing drug in schizophrenia, alcoholism and migraine, combined with vitamin C. Niacin also shares an antioxidant effect with other members of the B complex vitamins.

The RDA for niacin is 18mg per day, but more is needed by men, pregnant women and breast-feeding women. More niacin is required by the body if the vitamins B_1 (thiamin), B_2 (riboflavin) and B_6 (pyridoxine) are deficient as these vitamins help in the conversion of tryptophan to niacin. The formation of niacin would seem to be inhibited by contraceptive pills. Two-thirds of the niacin we use is produced from tryptophan in the diet. Deficiency in niacin produces a wide range of symptoms, including muscle weakness, fatigue, loss of appetite, skin eruptions, irritability, nausea, vomiting, recurring headaches, tension, depression and insomnia. Severe niacin deficiency results in a disease called pellagra, which still occurs in slum areas of developed countries, in developing countries and in alcoholics. The characteristics include scaly dermatitis, inflammation of the mucous membranes, diarrhoea and mental disturbances that can include depression, confusion, delirium, disorientation and dementia. Ultimately, without niacin supplementation, the sufferer will die.

vitamin B_5

pantothenic acid, pantothenate

Pantothenic acid is a water-soluble vitamin that is required by most higher organisms for efficient functioning of the body. The structure of pantothenic acid was isolated in 1940 by J. R. Williams, who named the vitamin pantothenate. Vitamin B_5 is quite heat-resistant and is not destroyed by frying, cooking or baking, but it is lost in food cooked in a pressure cooker (because of the high temperatures) and in deep-frozen meat. Pantothenic acid is found in almost all foods, including beans, eggs, liver, whole-grain cereals, oranges, peanuts, wheat germ and fish. It is produced in the human gut by intestinal bacteria, but this does not meet the total amount of pantothenic acid required by the body. Pantothenic acid from the diet is absorbed in the stomach and small intestine, but very little vitamin B_5 is stored in the body, and it generally passes through the body unaltered. It is eliminated in the urine and excreta.

Pantothenic acid is essential for the metabolism of sugars, fats and proteins, as it forms part of co-enzyme A. This co-enzyme plays a very important role in the transfer of acetyl groups from various compounds in the Krebs cycle. Vitamin B_5 is also important in the formation and growth of new cells that are required for healthy skin and hair, and in the production of essential fatty acids. It is needed for the normal functioning of the steroid hormone cortisone, and it allows the body to use the vitamin-like substances choline and para-aminobenzoic acid

(PABA). Pantothenic acid's most important role is in the functioning of the B-lymphocytes, which are critical for the production of antibodies. Thus pantothenic acid plays a large role in cell defence against disease. As co-enzyme A, pantothenic acid is distributed throughout all body tissues, concentrating in the liver, heart and kidneys where large quantities of energy are required for proper functioning of the tissue. The blood levels of vitamin B_5 are usually between 100 and 400g per litre, and the RDA for vitamin B_5 is 10mg.

Vitamin B_5 deficiency is exceedingly rare in humans, and generally is found only in experimental conditions where volunteers are given a pantothenic acid-free diet. Under these conditions, symptoms that are seen include asthma, muscle cramps, insomnia, fatigue, stomach pain, numbness in the limbs, personality changes, discomfort, reduced antibody production, and increased susceptibility to allergy and infection. These problems are rectified by taking a supplement of pantothenic acid.

Pantothenic acid is also important in other species, e.g. birds and rats. In chickens, a lack of vitamin B_5 causes dermatitis and nerve degeneration in the spinal cord, and pantothenic acid is known as chick anti-dermatitis factor. In rats that are given pantothenic acid-free diets, the body hair loses pigmentation and turns grey. This effect has been reversed in some cases and pigmentation was returned to the hair. This occurrence did not provide firm evidence of a link between hair pigmentation and pantothenic acid in the diet in rats, and there is no evidence that a similar effect could occur in humans.

Salts of pantothenic acid have been used to treat various medical disorders. Sodium and potassium salts are used to help circulatory problems in the legs, including 'restless legs'. The calcium salt has been a good therapy for a condition called paralytic ileus in which a patient is unable to move for a long time after an operation. The salt is generally administered as an injection, with a very high dose of up to 1000mg being given. The vitamin aids the system as it improves the activity and peristalsis of the small intestine. Pantothenic acid ointments may be used to treat skin injuries and burns.

Most people will receive sufficient vitamin B_5 through their diet and supplements should not be required.

vitamin B_6

pyridoxine, pyridoxal, pyridoxamine, $C_8H_{11}NO_3$

Pyridoxine is a white, crystalline vitamin that forms part of the B complex group. It is water-soluble and was first isolated in its crystalline form in 1938. The precise structure of vitamin B_6 was deduced by Richard Kuhn in 1939. Pyridoxal and pyridoxamine are both related compounds with similar activity to the B_6 compound pyridoxine. In some species of bacteria the term pyridoxamine is preferred as the B_6 vitamin. Vitamin B_6 is required by most animals and bacteria species. The vitamin is found in many foods, including green vegetables, brewer's yeast, fish, pulses, milk, meat, liver, whole-grain cereals, nuts, raisins and prunes.

The vitamin has a very large range of actions in the body. Vitamin B_6 is essential for maintaining healthy skin and nerves, in the formation of red blood cells, in providing general resistance to disease, and to stop premature ageing. When taken into the body, pyridoxine is absorbed through the intestines and is rapidly metabolized and dispersed through the tissues. Monitoring of levels of vitamin B_6 can be done using whole blood, red blood cells or blood plasma, as they all reflect the patient's pyridoxine status. RDA values for vitamin B_6 are 2mg for women and 2.2mg for men. Greater B_6 requirements are seen in pregnant and breast-feeding women, people on a high protein diet, including athletes, people with chronic diseases, women on the contraceptive pill, and people with intestinal diseases, e.g. gluten allergy. In studies in Finland, up to 30 per cent of elderly residents in nursing homes were found to be deficient in vitamin B_6. The major functions of this vitamin include enzyme reactions, the formation of brain hormones, the formation of haemoglobin, and the maintenance of the homoeostatic balance of sodium and potassium ions in the body. Pyridoxine forms part of the pyridoxal diophosphate chemical, which is a prosthetic group associated with transamination reactions occurring in the mitochondria or cytosol of a cell. The chemical is important in allowing transaminase enzymes to function effectively, when they catalyse the conversion of alpha-amino acids into slightly different alpha-keto acids. This process is very important in the breakdown and synthesis of amino acids in the body. Vitamin B_6 is important in allowing the conversion of tryptophan in the diet into vitamin B_3 (niacin) and in the breakdown of glucose to a different form—glucose-1-phosphate—in the glycolysis process.

The vitamin is known to promote formation of hormones that are important in brain function, to encourage proper absorption of vitamin B_{12} (cyanocobalamin), to help the body utilize magnesium, and to be involved in the production of hydrochloric acid in the stomach. Vitamin B_6 improves the activity of both Band T-lymphocytes in our immune system, and this in turn helps to prevent diseases such as asthma, arthritis, cancer, coronary heart disease, various allergies and circulatory disorders. It regulates the ionic balance between sodium and potassium ions, allows proper uptake and use of the mineral selenium in the body, and partially controls the functioning and repair of the nervous and musculo-skeletal systems. Pyridoxine is essential for the formation of the haem group in haemoglobin, and it may also act to reduce the cholesterol level in the blood. The production of antibodies occurs because of vitamin B_6, and it also acts to stop aggregation of blood platelets in blood vessels, which commonly cause blood clots. The vitamin may provide protection against arteriosclerosis and heart attacks as it prevents the formation of plaque in artery walls. This occurrence has been seen in studies of monkeys and rabbits, and it is now confirmed in humans. Indeed, the action of vitamin B_6 resembles the action of essential fatty acids, in that deficiency symptoms are similar, and these symptoms can be cured using supplements of either substance. The precise mechanism for these beneficial effects of vitamin B_6 and EFAs are not known.

In some cases of acute heart attack, investigation showed that the patients had low levels of vitamin B_6 in their bodies. Some people have an hereditary condition that means they need an increased daily intake of vitamin B_6. This generally appears in the first few months after birth when the vitamin-deficient baby may suffer from epilepsy-like convulsions, but these frightening symptoms can be removed by pyridoxine supplementation. Deficiency in vitamin B_6 can result in loss of appetite, anaemia, emaciation, depression, fatigue, general apathy, nervousness, insomnia and poor memory. Symptoms can also include atrophy of the skin epidermis, hair follicles and sebaceous glands, oral cavity infections, hacks in the corners of the mouth, and a loss of the sense off touch in the limbs. These symptoms may indicate that other B vitamins are deficient from the diet, e.g. B_2 and B_{12}. Children and infants are more at risk from pyridoxine deficiency, when they can suffer from irritability, convulsions and anaemia.

For women, vitamin B_6 deficiency may be associated with discomfort and pain during menstruation and pregnancy. Lack of pyridoxine can be found in people with a high alcohol consumption, in women on the contraceptive pill, in elderly people and pregnant women. Vitamin B_6 can help to stabilize the blood/sugar balance during pregnancy and possibly to prevent the onset of diabetes during pregnancy.

Some medicines such as penicillamine (to prevent arthritis) and some tuberculosis medicines are antagonistic to vitamin B_6 and counteract its effects. This can lead to deficiency symptoms like drowsiness, convulsions and difficulty in walking. These problems can be resolved with supplements of 30–100mg per day in most cases, but symptoms related to the nervous system may only be stopped with a dosage of between 300 and 600mg per day. As a therapeutic remedy, pyridoxine is given to patients with intestinal diseases, cancer, asthma and after major intestinal surgery at a dose of 50–150mg. Angina pectoris can be treated with between 100 and 300mg of B_6 per day, as can people recovering after a heart attack. This can be of particular benefit when combined with the mineral selenium, as the two nutrients act to reduce blood platelet accumulation, and the chances of blood clots are also reduced. Vitamin B_6 can be of great benefit to asthma sufferers, especially when given along with antioxidants and essential fatty acids. Very large doses of more than 1000mg can be dangerous and cause poisoning and damage to the peripheral nervous system, including disturbing the sense of touch. Vitamin B_6 is also given as a supplement to ease painful periods, premenstrual syndrome and in endometriosis.

vitamin B_9

folic acid, folate, vitamin B_9, folacin; pteroyl-L-glutamic acid, $C_{19}N_7O_6H_{14}$

Folic acid is a water-soluble vitamin, which has a yellow crystalline structure. In humans, a small amount is produced by intestinal bacteria, but this may not be sufficient. It was discovered by Dr Lucy Wills in 1931 while she was researching into a form of anaemia in India. She found that the addition of yeast to the patient's diet cured the anaemia, and folic acid was finally isolated in 1941. The name folic acid is from the Latin folicum for 'leaf', as the vitamin was isolated from spinach leaves. Indeed, spinach, asparagus, green vegetables, liver, yeast, kidneys, nuts and whole grains are among the best natural sources of folic acid. The role of vitamin B_9 in our bodies is as a precursor of tetrahydrafolic acid, which is a co-enzyme that transfers single carbon groups in enzyme reactions. This allows the formation of purines and pyrimidines, which are essential to the formation of nucleic acids such as DNA (deoxyribonucleic acid). New nucleic acids are made when new cells are being produced, and hence folic acid is required to produce red blood cells and in new cell synthesis in tissue repair. The co-enzyme also allows the formation of the amino acids serine and glycine. This enzymatic role of vitamin B_9 occurs in conjunction with vitamin B_{12} (cyanocobalamin), and they are both required in rapidly dividing cells for protein and nucleic acid formation. Vitamin C is also involved in the formation of the haem grouping in haemoglobin, like vitamin B_6 pyridoxine.

Vitamin B_9 is also said to increase the appetite and stimulates production of hydrochloric acid in the digestive system. Some sources state that folic acid may help protect women against cervical dysplasia, which are precancerous changes in the cells of the uterine cervix. Folic acid and its derivatives are very important to the formation of new cells and hence to the growth and development of the human embryo. The normal RDA for folic acid is 400μg, and both prior to and during pregnancy, women should have around 800μg folic acid per day to help prevent dietary deficiencies that may lead to neural tube defects in the embryo, e.g. spina bifida. Women who have previously given birth to a child with a neural tube defect, or if there is a family history of children with neural tube defects, then the women should be placed on supplements of 4mg per day. Mouth deformities such as a cleft palate or hair lip may also be caused by folic acid deficiency during pregnancy. Folic acid is passed on to a newborn baby via a mother's breast milk.

Folic acid deficiency can occur in many people, and it is said to be the commonest vitamin deficiency in the world. Up to 45 per cent of people may be low in vitamin B_9, and it is a particular problem in elderly people. The vitamin is rapidly destroyed by cooking, so maintaining an adequate intake can be a problem in hospital or institutional environments where food is kept warm for a period of time with a subsequent loss in vitamin levels. Folic acid in the diet is absorbed through the small intestine, and some cycling from the bile back to the intestine occurs. Thus any problems in production of bile upsets the folic acid balance in the body. Humans hold very small reserves of folic acid in the body, and the folic acid balance can be monitored via whole blood, red blood cells or blood serum tests. Deficiency in vitamin B_9 is seen in people with high alcohol consumption, in elderly people on inadequate diets, in pregnant women, in women on contraceptive pills, and in people who fast. Problems with the intestine can lead to malabsorption of food and vitamins with possible deficiency symptoms. Too little folic acid can lead to the development of megaloblastic anaemia, which covers several types of anaemia, including pernicious anaemia. This disease was previously fatal until it was discovered in 1926 that the disease was caused by the malabsorption of vitamin B_{12} (cyanocobalamin). These megaloblastic anaemias occur in 20 per cent of expectant mothers and can also be seen in children. Insufficient folic acid has been found in 24 per cent of surgical hospital patients in Britain, where the deficiency produced symptoms of depression, apathy, oral cavity infections, respiratory problems, dizziness and grey coloration to the skin. Vitamin B_9 and its absorption in the body is adversely affected by epilepsy medicines such as phenytoin or phenobarbital. Long-term loss of appetite or chronic diseases like gluten allergy can mean there is insufficient folic acid intake with possible deficiency problems such as forgetfulness, confusion, insomnia, shortness of breath, irritability and weakness.

Several medicines are antagonistic to folic acid, such as drugs that treat cancer or urinary system complaints. These can prevent the proper use of vitamin B_9 and create deficiency symptoms. As a remedy, folic acid supplements can be taken by patients with anaemia and rheumatoid arthritis. In people who have had surgical removal of their stomach, careful monitoring of levels of folic acid and cyanocobalamin is required to maintain their health.

vitamin B_{12}

cyanocobalamin, cyanocobalamine, $C_{63}H_9OCoN_{14}O_{14}P$
Vitamin B_{12} is a water-soluble vitamin that contains cobalt, a cyanide group, and a nucleotide in its structure. It is dark red in colour with a crystalline structure, and was first isolated in 1948. The action of vitamin B_{12} is linked to vitamin B_9 (folic acid) and insufficient supplies of either causes deficiency symptoms. Cyanocobalamin forms part of the vitamin

B complex, and it is found in animal food sources, e.g. liver, fish, eggs, meat, kidney, dairy products (particularly cheese), fortified cereals and brewer's yeast. Vitamin B_{12} is absorbed only from the gastrointestinal tract in the presence of the intrinsic factor, which is a glycoprotein produced by the intestinal epithelium. Without the intrinsic factor and calcium, the vitamin cannot be absorbed through the intestinal mucous membranes and enter the bloodstream. The resulting vitamin deficiency can cause pernicious anaemia, brain damage and degeneration of the nervous system. Until the 20th century, pernicious anaemia had no known cause, and it always produced fatal results. In 1926 G. R. Minot and W. P. Murphy found that the disease could be treated with liver, and this introduced the critical factor required for red blood cell production into the body. This extrinsic factor essential for the formation of red blood cells is vitamin B_{12}. Today, people with pernicious anaemia need to take vitamin B_{12}, normally in the form of injections, every three months for the rest of their lives. Deficiency of B_{12} affects nearly all the tissues of the body, particularly those with rapidly dividing cells, e.g. bone marrow and gamete production. Other actions of cyanocobalamin include influencing the activity of B- and T-lymphocytes, acting on neural function, and in the biosynthesis of the amino acid methionine and the vitamin-like substance choline. A chemical called 5–deoxyadenosyl cobalamin has co-enzyme activity and is required to synthesize nucleotides, to maintain the protein myelin surrounding the nerves, to allow correct erythrocyte maturation and to permit the correct functioning of folic acid (vitamin B_9) in the body. The co-enzyme form also works in protein formation, in preventing cell degeneration and in the metabolism of fats, carbohydrates and proteins to produce energy.

Deficiency of vitamin B_{12} does not only cause pernicious anaemia but it also produces tongue infections, disturbances of the nervous system such as loss of sensation and poor coordination. Continuing lack of cyanocobalamin produces fatigue, irritability, loss of appetite, diarrhoea, stomach complaints, problems with the circulation and heart with the skin colour becoming yellow. Menstrual disturbances, an unpleasant body odour, neuritis and numbness or tingling in the hands and feet may occur in a sufferer. Symptoms of pernicious anaemia can include additional mental problems such as loss of concentration, depression, paranoia and irritation. Many people with this disease show changes in the pattern of electrical impulses in the brain, which may be because of damaged myelin in the nerve endings. An interesting point is that 2 per cent of all psychiatric patients suffer from pernicious anaemia.

vitamin B_{15}

pangamate, pangamic acid

Whether this substance is a vitamin or provitamin is the subject of great debate. It was first isolated from apricot kernels in 1951, and it is also found in rice husks, horse liver, ox blood, brewer's yeast, maize and other plants. It was discovered by E. T. Krebs, who is said to have believed that pangamate has all-powerful properties. The chemical name for pangamate is glucono-dimethyl acetylate, and it is proposed to be a cure for alcoholism, hepatitis, cancer, diabetes and other diseases as well as being an antidote to toxins. Active research into the compound has been carried out in the former Soviet Union, but most government agencies, e.g. American Food and Drug Administration (FDA), do not believe there is enough evidence to show this substance is beneficial to health.

vitamin B$_{17}$

amygdalin, laetrile, C$_{20}$H$_{27}$NO$_{11}$

This substance is a naturally occurring glycoside that is found in most fruits of the Rosaceae family, particularly almonds and apricots. The reputation of this compound is better than that of pangamate, but it is unsure whether amygdalin is a vitamin or not. The substance has the chemical formula C$_{20}$H$_{27}$NO$_{11}$, which includes a C=N cyanide group, and it can be hydrolysed to produce benzaldehyde, glucose and hydrogen cyanide. Some sources suggest that amygdalin has a cancer-preventative effect. In some cases, amygdalin is taken by people to treat cancer only when they are on a diet that may help prevent cancer. The diet is mostly fruit and nuts with very high doses of minerals. The anti-cancer effects are said to be because of the production of hydrogen cyanide (HCN) in the tissues, which attacks and destroys cancer cells. Unfortunately, the hydrogen cyanide also kills healthy cells and is one of the most potent poisons known to man. Studies to try and determine the effects of amygdalin have had conflicting results, but many researchers now believe that amygdalin can cause cyanide poisoning or even cancer. Laetrile is the trade name given to amygdalin, and there may still be some limited use for amygdalin in alterative medicine.

vitamin C

ascorbic acid

Vitamin C is a white crystalline vitamin that was first isolated in 1932 by Charles Glen King. It was first synthesized artificially in 1933 by Tadeus Reichstein. It is water-soluble but is easily destroyed by cooking and contact with alkalis, and it can be easily oxidized. Ascorbic acid is also lost to some degree if food is deep-frozen or preserved. It is present in citrus fruit, berries, tomatoes, fresh green vegetables, potatoes, peppers, broccoli, cauliflower, some fruit juices and chillies. For healthy adults, an RDA of 60mg is recommended, with pregnant women requiring a higher intake. This intake would allow reserves of around 1500mg to build up in the body. An increased daily intake is needed for smokers, people on contraceptive pills or living in very hot or very cold environments. In Scandinavia, for example, deficiency diseases of vitamin C, such as scurvy, are still a problem in the long winter months as the body's reserves become depleted and there is little in the way of fresh fruit and vegetables to replace the body's stored supply. Various problems can arise from lack of vitamin C, depending upon the severity of the deficiency. The most severe disease is scurvy, which was common among sailors in the days of sailing ships, when fresh fruit and vegetables were not available on a long voyage and vitamin depletion occurred. Symptoms of scurvy start with swelling, inflammation and bleeding of the gums, often with loss of teeth, followed by haemorrhages under the skin, muscular weakness and serious joint damage because of haemorrhages. Over time, the disease causes anaemia, mouth ulceration and induration of the leg muscles. Milder deficiencies show up as tender joints, bleeding or soft gums, fatigue, weakness, reduced immunity to infections, irritability and muscle degeneration.

These deficiency problems illustrate that vitamin C is essential for the formation of collagen and connective tissues, and for production of the fibrous material found in the intercellular matrices in bone and teeth. Collagen is used for the formation of skin ligaments, tendons and cartilage. Ascorbic acid is also important for maintaining the strength of capillary walls and for aiding the absorption of iron, and it is needed to produce stress hormones. Vitamin C also improves resistance to infection and helps fight diseases such as high blood pressure, cancer and arteriosclerosis. Ascorbic acid is known to act as a co-factor in the oxidation of the amino acid tyrosine, and it may take part in oxidation-reduction reactions in energy metabolism.

Like many other vitamins and minerals, vitamin C has protective properties if taken in larger doses. Vitamin C is an antioxidant and, more importantly, it has a reinforcing influence in the period of activity and effects of other antioxidants, e.g. vitamins A and E. These three vitamins have a synergistic relationship, in that they increase each other's effects in the body. Ascorbic acid has a particularly important function in the brain as it protects against the effects of ischaemia or oxygen deficiency. This deficiency and the subsequent reperfusion of the area produce oxygen-free radicals that can destroy cells. In the body, the highest levels of vitamin C are to be found in nerve tissues and the brain, which are those most at risk from free radical damage.

This beneficial antioxidant action of vitamin C can be reversed if the vitamin itself is oxidized. When vitamin C is exposed to light, heat or air, a chemical called dehydroascorbate (DHA) is formed. This substance has a completely different effect from vitamin C—it is a pro-oxidant that encourages the production of oxygen-free radicals, leading to cell damage. Oxidation of vitamin C also occurs when it contacts iron or copper within the food. Mainly, the vitamin is protected by the cell membranes, but if they are removed by cooking then the vitamin C is attacked by the metals and is lost or transformed to dehydroascorbate.

Vitamin C, like vitamin A and selenium, is thought to be able to prevent the formation and development of cancer. When taken in large doses, vitamin C can prevent nitrites and nitrates in our foodstuffs from being converted into nitrosamines. Most of these nitrosamines are carcinogenic and can lead to the development of stomach cancer or cancer of the intestinal tract. This cancer-preventing action may extend to cancer of the throat or womb and malignant melanomas.

A further protective effect of vitamin C is that the vitamin improves the function of white blood cells called phagocytes. The role of the phagocytes in humans is to find, destroy and consume viruses, bacteria and cancer cells. Vitamin C also activates white blood cells called neutrophils and increases the level of antibodies found in the blood, in connection with elevated levels of the cellular protein interferon, which attacks viruses.

Ascorbic acid can help to prevent or lessen allergic reactions as it inhibits the action of histamine. Histamine is normally released when there is an allergic reaction in the respiratory passages, the skin or in the mucous membranes in the nose, and can lead to itching, rash formation, runny nose and breathing difficulties. Thus, vitamin C can lessen these symptoms and help in self-treatment of allergies. In some rare cases, vitamin C itself can trigger an allergic reaction.

Vitamin C acts along with vitamin B_1 (thiamin) and the amino acid cysteine to prevent the chemicals formalin, formaldehyde and acetaldehyde causing damage to the body. These harmful chemicals are produced by the breakdown of alcohol in the body or by tobacco smoke. Other chemicals that vitamin C acts against include nicotine, nitrogen compounds, vehicle exhaust fumes, and the toxic heavy metal cadmium. This explains why alcoholics or smokers have much lower levels of vitamin C in their blood, as it is consumed by these toxic substances. Supplements of vitamin C, selenium, zinc, beta-carotene, vitamins A and E and ubiquinone may help counterbalance some of the harmful effects of smoking.

Another vital protective role of vitamin C is in protecting heart muscle after a heart attack. Research has found that the white blood cells transport large quantities of vitamin C from other parts of the body to the heart. This could mean that other tissues become deficient in vitamin C, and blood levels could fall without adequate vitamin C supplementation. Vitamin C has the same role when the coronary arteries undergo hardening and narrow. Ascorbic acid also prevents and repairs cell damage in the blood vessels of the heart, and intravenous injections of vitamin C can reduce the chances of blood platelet aggregation, hence reducing the risk of blood clots and arteriosclerosis.

Vitamin C may influence the balance between 'good' (HDL-) cholesterol and 'bad' (LDL-) cholesterol to increase levels of the HDL-cholesterol, and may be involved in preventing high blood pressure and arteriosclerosis, according to studies carried out in Finland. Large-scale research done by the World Health Organization showed that antioxidants, including vitamin C, inhibited the LDL-cholesterol from oxidizing into oxidized cholesterol, which forces itself into artery walls and is involved in the formation of arteriosclerosis. So vitamin C can prevent dangerous forms of cholesterol developing and reduces levels of the LDL-cholesterol.

Supplements of vitamin C normally cause few problems, but doses of several grams per day can lead to stomach problems in some people. This can normally be avoided if a soluble vitamin C tablet is taken or if the supplement is taken after meals. It is best to work your way up gradually to a large dose of vitamin C, as sudden high intakes can cause diarrhoea. On the other hand, stopping large doses of vitamin C suddenly is not advisable as it can lead to feelings of fatigue. The dose taken each day should be reduced gradually if a person wishes to stop taking large doses of vitamin C.

vitamin D

D_2 ergocalciferol/calciferol, D_3 cholecaliferol
This vitamin is actually a related group of hormone-like chemicals called steroid alcohols. Vitamin D1 was the first to be discovered and turned out to be a crude mixture of steroid alcohols. Ergocalciferol is the name given to vitamin D_2, and it is produced from the provitamin ergosterol in plants. The conversion occurs because of the action of ultraviolet light on the chemical. Vitamin D_3 or cholecalciferol is derived from the provitamin dehydrocholesterol, which is widely distributed in the skin. When sunlight or ultraviolet light encounters the provitamin, it causes a change into the active form of it. In humans, vitamin D_3 may also be formed in milk when it is exposed to sunlight.

The group of vitamin D chemicals was first isolated as crystals in 1931. Both vitamins D_2 and D_3 are white, crystalline alcohols, and they differ only in the structure of their chemical side chains and in their melting points. These minor changes still mean that both forms have almost identical actions. Vitamin D is fat-soluble and is found in animal fats, butter, eggs, liver, fish (particularly kippers, mackerel, sardines and tuna), margarine, full-fat dairy products, malted milk drinks and evaporated milk. Milk is rich in vitamin D only if it is fortified. In the United States milk is fortified with 400 IU per litre while Germany adds 750–1000 IU of vitamin D per litre. Vitamin D in food is quite stable, and it is not lost through storage, processing or cooking. Fish liver oils are very rich sources of vitamins D and A, and the use of fish liver oils to cure deficiency diseases was first carried out in 1918. In bright sunlight, the skin can produce up to 10 IU of vitamin D_3 per square centimetre of skin, depending on the level of pigment in the skin. Dark skin allows less ultraviolet light to reach the deeper layers of the skin and so less vitamin D is produced. Air pollution, which absorbs ultraviolet light, can also reduce the penetration of ultraviolet rays into the skin and lessen the level of vitamin D produced. Like vitamin A, the recommended requirements for vitamin D are set in IU. Supplements of 1000 IU per day are recommended for infants between two weeks and two years of age. Then from two years to fifteen years, supplements of 500–1000 IU should be given daily. The adult RDA is around 400 IU, while nursing mothers are recommended to consume between 400 and 800 IU daily. Supplements of vitamin D are generally required only in the dark winter months, particularly for children and elderly people.

Humans absorb vitamin D through the small intestine, with bile involved in the process. Hence diseases of the pancreas, liver, gall bladder or intestines can reduce vitamin D absorption, as can disruption to the absorption of fats or anti-epilepsy medication. Monitoring the level of vitamin D in the body can be done by analysing blood serum, as vitamin D binds itself to certain blood proteins. The form produced is 25–dihydroxycholecalciferol, and this is produced in the liver from calciferol. Vitamin D has various effects on the body. It acts like a hormone and has effects on distant areas of the body. The vitamin acts on the body to aid the absorption of calcium and phosphorus from the ileum into the blood, which are then used in the formation and strengthening of bones and teeth. Deleterious effects can occur with large doses of vitamin D, as if too much phosphorus and calcium are present in the blood, the bones and teeth can become over-calcified, calculus stones may form in the kidneys and other organs, and hardening of the arteries, because of calcium deposits, may occur. If supplement intake is in excess of 50,000 IU daily, there is a risk of overdose, and by taking 25,000 IU daily over a long period, poisoning can occur. Symptoms of this extreme intake are general discomfort, itchy eyes and skin, unquenchable thirst, and frequent diarrhoea. Also, tests would show calcium build-up in the blood vessels, liver, lungs and kidneys. Because of these severe symptoms and the risk of overdose, adults should take only around 400 IU per day. The other role of vitamin D is to regulate the permeability of cell membranes.

Deficiency of vitamin D causes rickets in children, with irregular growth and softening of the bones. It can also lead to distorted limbs, swollen joints and deformities of the chest. Rickets is still seen in children of some developing countries but is rare in the industrialized world. A similar disease called osteomalacia occurs in adults, where calcium is lost from the bone matrix, making it soft with accompanying weakness, fracture, pain and weight loss. This may be particularly common during pregnancy. In children, vitamin D is essential to the normal development of teeth, and lack of vitamin D can give rise to dental caries. In both children and adults, lack of vitamin D and reduced levels of calcium in the blood may prompt muscle weakness and cramp, as the calcium is needed for correct contraction and relaxation of both smooth muscle and cardiac muscle tissue. With extended periods of vitamin D deficiency, which has led to reduced calcium absorption, a disease called osteoporosis can occur. Here the body reabsorbs existing bone so that the quantity of bone mass is reduced. It causes pain, particularly in the lower back, with loss of stature and an increased risk of fractures. The disease may occur naturally in post-menopausal women, in immobilized patients, in long-term steroid treatments and because of extreme vitamin D/calcium deficiency.

vitamin E

tocopherols–alpha, beta, gamma and delta (α, β, γ and δ) forms
This vitamin is actually a group of closely related compounds, all of which have vitamin E activity. They are fat-soluble, and the strongest and most commonly used chemical is alpha-tocopherol. They cannot be produced in the human body, and we depend entirely on our dietary intake. Good sources of vitamin E are wheat germ, soya bean, cotton seed, corn and peanut oils, margarine, raw seeds and nuts, eggs, butter, sweet potatoes, liver and some green-leaved vegetables. Unfortunately, much of the vitamin E in foodstuffs is lost because of contact with the air, processing, preserving and deep-freezing. Vitamin E was first discovered in 1923, when experiments on rats showed that a lack of vitamin E caused infertility in male rats and an increased risk of miscarriage in female rats. Further study found that similar reproductive problems arose in other vertebrate groups, along with kidney degeneration and other wasting symptoms.

The role of vitamin E in the body includes being essential for muscle development, and it is important in making red blood cells resistant to haemolysis or breakdown. It may also be essential for normal reproductive function in both sexes, but the precise mechanism for this process is as yet unknown. The most important action vitamin E has is as a lipid-soluble antioxidant that protects highly unsaturated fatty acids in cell membranes from attack by free radicals and peroxides. It acts inside the cell to maintain the stability of polyunsaturated fatty acids and similar fat-like compounds, such as hormones from the pituitary, adrenal and sex glands, as well as vitamin A. The antioxidant properties of vitamin E are enhanced by the enzyme glutathione peroxidase, which contains selenium. Vitamin C is also important in prolonging and reinforcing the beneficial effects of vitamin E.

Counting Calories

As an antioxidant, vitamin E has recently shown that, in connection with selenium, it can prevent cancer in experimental animals. Further research has told us that vitamin E may be of use as a prophylactic drug for cancer in humans and can also help patients undergoing radiotherapy or chemotherapy withstand the treatment, with less harmful side effects. Indeed, blood serum values of vitamin E of less than 18 μmol l^{-1} have been shown to suggest an increased risk of cancer. Another area of interest is that of cardiovascular diseases and blood clots, and how vitamin E can help these conditions. How vitamin E works in the body would seem to be connected to prostaglandins, but research into this link has only just started. High doses of vitamin E are known to stop the aggregation of blood platelets and so help prevent blood clots or thromboses forming. At megadoses greater than 800mg per day, vitamin E acts as an anticoagulant that prevents or delays blood clotting. Since the 1940s vitamin E has been used for correcting cardiovascular disorders like claudicatio intermittens (window-watcher's disease). This disease causes sufferers to struggle to walk even short distances because of a circulatory disorder in the legs, and many patients found supplements of vitamin E very helpful. The only drawback is that it may take several to many months for a beneficial effect to arise.

Patients with coronary heart disease who are treated with vitamin E show conflicting results Some studies in the early days of vitamin E treatment showed very good results, but more recent research has been disappointing. Vitamin E influences the development and functioning of the smooth and striped muscles, and is able to prevent muscle degeneration. It is particularly good for cardiac muscles. However, a new water-soluble analogue of vitamin E has been manufactured, and this has been shown in animal studies to have a good protective effect on the heart. Best results are obtained with the new vitamin E analogue, selenium and vitamin E itself. Like vitamins A, B$_5$, B$_6$ and C, vitamin E improves the activity of the immune system and so strengthens resistance to diseases, including those of a bacterial or viral nature. In order for this to occur, supplements in the range of 5–20mg per kilogram of body weight are required, which works out at 350–1400mg for a person weighing 70kg (154lbs). Vitamin E also acts to prevent cataract formation, when daily doses of 300–400mg are taken. This effect is reinforced by beta-carotene and vitamin C. This vitamin also protects against overdoses of selenium and digoxin, a heart stimulant obtained from the foxglove plant. Vitamin E may also have detoxifying effects on the side effects of cytostatic drugs like adriamycin and may detoxify harmful heavy metals such as cadmium.

One of the most promising areas of vitamin E therapy is in Parkinson's disease, which is a progressive, degenerative, neurological disorder caused by damage in the cerebral ganglia and lack of neurotransmitters. It is more common in men, normally developing in people over sixty, and with no known cure. Most treatments try to keep the condition under control but with limited success. Ongoing research in Canada and the United States has shown that the disease may occur because of the action of free radicals, suggesting that antioxidants may be of benefit in preventing the illness in the first place. This study has also shown that doses of 300mg of vitamin C and of 400–3200mg of vitamin E per day could slow down the progress of the disease. Indeed, antioxidant vitamin therapy could delay the requirement for traditional Parkinson's medicines such as levo-dopa. These large daily doses of vitamin C and E caused no problems with no signs of toxicity. Vitamin E is also recommended for heart patients with angina pectoris or recent heart attack patients at a dose of 400mg each day, often in association with other antioxidants and selenium. Doses of up to 1000mg per day are used to prevent new blood clots and to improve the heart muscle's resistance to oxygen deficiency. This vitamin is important for women as it can be taken during pregnancy and when breast-feeding with no risk of harm to the baby. Vitamin E is vital for both male and female fertility and prevents miscarriage of the foetus as it promotes the normal development of the foetus in the womb and ensures a normal pregnancy without complications. Vitamin E may also be given as a therapy in rheumatism and at the menopause. Unfortunately, attempts to use vitamin E to help some muscle diseases and muscular dystrophy have not had many beneficial results. Elderly people can benefit from supplements of vitamin E and selenium. Studies in Germany and Finland have shown that 400mg of vitamin E per day results in a significant improvement in the psychological and physical health of elderly people.

Like the other fat-soluble vitamins, vitamin E is stored in the body, but there is no risk of overdosing. Studies completed in Canada have shown that doses of up to 10g of vitamin E per day over an extended time gave rise to no ill effects. Some people, however, taking doses of 1000mg and more a day may develop stomach problems and diarrhoea.

vitamin H

biotin

Debate continues as to whether biotin is classified as a vitamin or as one of the B complex vitamins. Biotin was identified in 1940 by Albert Szent-Györgyi, Vincent Du Vigneaud and co-workers. It is water-soluble, crystalline and lacking in colour when isolated. The vitamin is found in liver, kidney, egg yolk, yeast, oats, nuts, milk chocolate and most vegetables. It is also produced naturally by intestinal bacteria, and this normally covers most of our daily requirements. Deficiency may result if a person consumes large quantities of raw egg white. The egg white contains a glycoprotein, called avidin, that forms a complex with biotin that cannot be broken down by the digestive enzymes. This only really occurs if around 20 raw egg whites are consumed per day, and this is fairly uncommon today.

Biotin is an active compound that participates in many enzymatic reactions. It serves as a prosthetic group on the enzyme, which fixes carbon dioxide into an organic compound. This occurs in intermediate compounds in the Krebs cycle, which produces energy from dietary glucose. Biotin is also known as a co-enzyme in the synthesis of fatty acids and purines in the body. Unusually, biotin is also involved in gluconeogenesis, a process in which glucose is produced from non-carbohydrate sources, e.g. amino acids. This occurs only when the diet contains insufficient carbohydrate for energy needs. Biotin also contributes to the production of antibodies and increases the effectiveness of the immune system.

Deficiency of biotin can occur and produces symptoms of loss of appetite, infections of the mucous membranes, depression, insomnia, muscle pains, rashes, discomfort and increased levels of cholesterol in the blood. These problems can be cleared up easily by daily injections of 150–300μg of biotin. Elderly people, athletes and people with epilepsy are known to have relatively low levels of biotin in their blood. Children may be affected by two skin diseases that have been linked to biotin deficiency. Leiner's disease is a widespread form of seborrhoeic eczema linked to lack of biotin, while the other is a more serious fungoid infection. This infection affects the growth of hair and causes disorders of both the central nervous system and the immune system. This all stems from a malfunction of the carboxylase enzyme, which requires biotin to function effectively, and it is resolved within a few days of biotin supplementation. Fortunately, both diseases are exceedingly rare.

Biotin has been tried as part of a therapy to stop hair loss. Combinations of 200–400μg of biotin, para-aminobenzoic acid (PABA), inositol, minerals and essential fatty acids have been tried with variable success.

vitamin K

K$_1$—phytomenadione, K$_2$—menaquinane, K$_3$—menadione
Vitamin K is a fat-soluble vitamin that exists in three forms. Vitamin K$_1$ is a yellow substance that is produced naturally in plants but has also been made artificially. Vitamin K$_2$ is a slightly less active form of compound with a pale yellow colour and a more unsaturated structure than K$_1$. It is synthesized by various microorganisms that live in the gastrointestinal tract in humans. Vitamin K$_3$ (menadione) is of synthetic origin and is of much less importance than the other forms. Vitamins K$_4$ and K$_5$ are also produced artificially. They have twice the biological effects of natural vitamin K (K$_1$ or K$_2$). Vitamin K, like vitamin E, exists as a group of similar chemicals, called quinones, which are essential for human health. Much of the vitamin K requirement is covered by

the vitamin K_2 produced by the intestinal bacteria. It is found in green vegetables, especially brassica species, seaweed, potatoes, liver, eggs, wheat germ, fish, nuts, alfalfa, molasses, yoghurt, fish liver oils, dairy products, corn and soya bean oils.

Vitamin K was discovered in 1935 by Henrik Dam, when he found that a mixture of alfalfa and putrefying fish powder could prevent haemorrhaging in chickens fed on a low-fat diet. The chemical isolated from alfalfa was phytomenadione—K_1. Vitamin K is resistant to heat, air and damp conditions, but the chemicals quickly decompose on exposure to sunlight or ultraviolet light. Like other fat-soluble vitamins, vitamin K is absorbed with fat in the intestines and then moves into the bloodstream via the lymphatic system.

The role of vitamin K in the body appears to be in allowing the synthesis of coagulation factors such as prothrombin in the liver. Prothrombin is found free in the blood and is the inactive precursor to thrombin itself. Thrombin is an enzyme coagulation factor that converts the soluble protein fibrinogen into the insoluble protein fibrin at the last stage of blood-clotting. Vitamin K is involved in the production of a number of coagulation factors, which, like prothrombin, undertake a series of reactions that turn blood from a liquid to a solid state, reducing blood loss and sealing the wound so that it may heal more successfully. Some sources believe that vitamin K is also involved in the electron transport chain and oxidative phosphorylation; two components of energy metabolism.

Deficiency in phytomenadione (vitamin K_1) may lead to the onset of osteoporosis or brittle bone disease. Vitamin K_1 is the catalyst for the metabolism of osteocalcin, which makes up the protein matrix for new bone formation. As long as vitamin K_1 is present, osteocalcin will bind calcium ions, and the bones will undergo calcification as normal. Many bone specialists now recommend monitoring the blood serum level of vitamin K_1 to check women at risk from osteoporosis and to try to prevent the disease starting. If osteoporosis is already affecting a woman's bones, then supplements of vitamin K_1 would give a better chance of recalcifying her bone tissues with fewer problems of pain, fractures or loss of stature. Blood serum testing is now recommended for women with the disease and women whose family history shows osteoporosis. This testing may not be possible in people on anticoagulant therapy after blood clotting or thrombosis problems. Deficiency in vitamin K_1 normally arises in people who do not eat enough green vegetables and in people whose digestion and absorption of fats is impaired. Studies in Japan have shown that supplements of vitamin K_1 in osteoporotic women reduced the calcium loss from their bones from 18 to 50 per cent and that vitamin K_1 supplements resulted in faster healing of bone fractures, both in normal and osteoporotic individuals.

Counting Calories

Deficiency of vitamin K can occur because of alcoholism, liver and intestinal diseases and in disturbances to fat absorption in the digestive system. Long-term antibiotic use may suppress the natural bacterial flora of the gastrointestinal tract producing vitamin K, so there is a risk of internal bleeding as the blood lacks the necessary coagulation factors.

Aspirin-containing painkillers also increase the body's requirement for vitamin K. Vitamin K is also given to patients before some types of major surgery, and it has been confirmed that large doses (more than 800mg) of vitamin E has an anticoagulant property that interferes with the addition of vitamin K. Supplements of vitamin K are generally given only as a preventative treatment to people at risk from osteoporosis, to osteoporotic people, to people with livers damaged by alcohol, or to people with severe burns who are treated with antibiotics. Newborn babies are given injections of vitamin K to prevent haemorrhage, as they do not have intestinal bacteria that produce it naturally until a few days after birth. People should consult their doctor before starting supplements of vitamin K, and some people with liver diseases cannot tolerate the action of the vitamin. There is no official RDA for vitamin K, but most adults require at least 1mg per day.

vitamin P

bioflavinoids, rutin, citrin, hesperidin

This name is given to a group of naturally occurring coloured pigments that are produced by plants. They are generally found in citrus fruits or vegetables as orange or yellow pigments. Bioflavinoids are found in carrots, rosehips, plums, oranges, lemons, etc, and the human requirement is thought to be very small. Bioflavinoids may be found as crystalline structures or as flavone glycosides in plants, depending on the type of bioflavinoid. They act in the body to strengthen the walls of blood capillaries and so prevent purpura, or bleeding into the tissues. Bioflavinoids are also known to be essential for the absorption and metabolism of vitamin C in the body. Supplements of bioflavinoids are taken by athletes, as they are suggested to heal pulled muscles faster and speed healing of sprained joints and chafed skin. Bioflavinoids may also be of benefit in treating hypertension (high blood pressure) and in reinforcing the beneficial effects of vitamin C on the connective tissues. Rutin ($C_{27}H_{30}O_{16}$, $3H_2O$) is a crystalline bioflavinoid found in buckwheat, which acts as an antioxidant. It is very well thought of in Russia, where diet supplements of 1g of rutin is given each day as a protective measure.

Vitamin-like Substances

carnitine

$(CH_3)_3 NCH_2 CH(OH) CH_2 COOH$

chemical name: alpha-hydroxy-gamma-butyo-betaine

This is a vitamin-like substance that is found in several tissues, including skeletal and heart muscle. It functions as a carrier molecule, moving fatty acids across the mitochondrial membrane inside cells. This allows biosynthesis of fatty acids or breakdown of the fatty acids to release energy. Carnitine can be synthesized in sufficient quantity in humans and higher animals, but its presence is required in the diet of some insects, including mealworms (Tenebrio species).

choline

$OHC_2H_4 N(CH_3)_3 OH$

chemical name: trimethyl-2-hydroxyethylammonium hydroxide

This is an alkaline compound that was first discovered in the 1930s. It was formerly classed as a B complex vitamin but is now termed a vitamin-like substance. It is found in wheat bran, egg yolk, brewer's yeast and offal, and only around 500mg of choline is required per day. This level is normally covered in vegetables, milk or lecithin intake. Choline is a constituent of a number of phospholipids, including lecithin (phosphatidylcholine), and also part of the neurotransmitter acetylcholine. For choline to be produced in humans requires an adequate supply of vitamin B_{12} (cyanocobalamin), vitamin B_9 (folic acid) and the amino acid methionine. It is still an essential vitamin for some animals and microorganisms.

Choline is involved in the synthesis of phospholipids, which form part of all lipid membranes, and is also involved with the transport of fats through the body. It is also essential for the metabolism of fats in humans and, apart from methionine, is the only substance known to take part in methylating reactions in the metabolism. It has been suggested that choline may reduce high levels of cholesterol in the blood, and it is possible that choline can pass over the blood brain barrier. Some studies indicate that it can improve the memory, but these claims have not been conclusively proven.

Deficiencies of choline in experiments with animals have caused fatty liver and cirrhosis of the liver, along with increased cholesterol levels, higher blood pressure and kidney damage. These results have not been repeated for humans. Choline deficiency has been linked to arterio-sclerosis and even Alzheimer's disease, where rapid ageing of the brain tissue occurs and the patient becomes prematurely senile.

Supplementation of the diet with choline has no real basis, and some forms of choline may adversely affect the activity of intestinal bacteria, interrupting production of other vitamins.

inositol

$C_6H_{12}O_6$
chemical name: hexahydroxycyclohexane

This compound is an isomer of glucose, which exists in nine stereo-iso-meric forms. The biologically active form is meso or i-inositor, which is widely distributed in plants and animals. Inositol is found in liver, wheat bran, maize (sweet corn), nuts, milk, brewer's yeast, oats, fruit, syrup, whole grains, cabbage, raisins, grapefruit, lecithin and peanuts. It is an essential vitamin and growth factor in some microorganisms and mice, but its exact function in the human body is unclear. Inositol was first isolated in the 1800s and is called a sugar alcohol because chemically it is an alcohol but its ring structure is similar to a sugar. In nature, inosi-tol exists in at least four forms in compounds or complexes with salts or metals. Meso-inositol is absorbed into the body through the intestines, from where it moves to the heart, other muscles, the brain and other organs. Some of it is also used in the glucose metabolism. Meso-inositol also acts as the precursor to a phosphoglyceride, called phosphatidyl inositol, which forms an important part of the membranes, muscles and brain. Experiments on animals have shown that inositol has similar effects to choline in that it takes part in the construction of cell mem-branes and plasma lipoproteins, and inositol inhibits the accumulation of fat in the liver and other organs. Inositol is also found in the urine of diabetic people in higher levels than normal.

Deficiencies of inositol have been carried out experimentally in mice, where they show loss of hair, rashes, constipation, reduced growth and milk secretion, and congenital eye defects. These conditions could not be related to human deficiency of the compound.

para-aminobenzoic acid (PABA)

$C_7H_7NO_2$
other name: 4-aminobenzoic acid (PAB)

This substance exists as yellowish-red crystals and is a component of the folic acid (vitamin B_9) molecule. It was formerly included in the group of B complex vitamins. PABA is produced from intestinal bacteria in humans and can be detected in human urine, blood, sweat and spinal fluid. It is also contained in meat, cereals, eggs and milk. The chemical can prevent the hair of experimental animals turning grey, and can even restore normal hair colour if it has been caused by deficiencies of vitamin H (biotin), vitamin B_9 (folic acid) or vitamin B_5 (pantothenic acid). This process does not occur in humans. PABA is very similar in its chemical structure to drugs known as sulphonamides, which replace PABA in the processing reactions of bacteria, so preventing the bacteria from maturing and reproducing. So care should be taken as PABA can counteract treatment with sulphonamides and in lotions or creams as a sunscreen. PABA is nontoxic except in very large doses when it can lead to vomiting and discomfort.

ubiquinone, co-enzyme Q/co-enzyme Q10

structure $Q_{10} = C_9O_4H_9–C_5OH_9O$ chain
This chemical consists of a substituted benzoquinone with a long hydrocarbon chain. The number of repeated C_5H_9 units attached to the benzoquinone core varies from species to species, with yeasts having six or seven units (co-enzyme Q_6 or Q_7), some bacteria having eight (co-enzyme Q_8), and humans having co-enzyme Q_{10} as the biologically active form. In humans, it is found in the heart muscle. Ubiquinone has an important role in the metabolism as it forms part of the electron transport chain in the mitochondria. Ubiquinone, along with the other eight chemicals that make up the electron transport chain, is embedded in the inner membrane of the mitochondrion where each chemical switches between a reduced and an oxidized state, and the whole process produces energy. Ubiquinone exists in the oxidized quinone and the reduced quinol form when it has been given electrons or hydrogen from the flavoprotein above it in the chain.

Ubiquinone also acts as an antioxidant in cells and is of particular benefit in protecting heart patients from reperfusion injury. It is given to many heart patients as a protective measure. In Japan, ubiquinone is registered as a medicine.

lecithin

phosphatidylcholine
This substance belongs to a group called phospholipids, which are essential for the formation of cell membranes. Lecithin has developed into a popular food supplement in recent years, and it is found in soya beans and vegetable oils. It is also produced naturally in the human body as it forms part of bile, the digestive liquid that helps to break down fats in our diet. Lecithin has a specific role that helps to make cholesterol soluble. The phosphoglyceride is found in all animal and vegetable cells, both in the cell membranes and in the motochondrial membranes. Indeed, 40 per cent of brain tissue is made of phosphatidyl choline, which is a form of lecithin. Lecithin contains both choline and

inositol in its structure, and this explains its large role in fat metabolism. Lecithin is also present in the lung surfactant, found in foetal and newborn lung tissue, that stops the walls of the lungs sticking together and collapsing. Several studies into the potential health benefits of lecithin have been carried out, and some people believe that lecithin may be able to decrease cholesterol levels and therefore reduce the risk of arteriosclerosis, ischaemic heart disease and blood clots. Similar research programmes have discovered that lecithin may improve the mental wellbeing and memory of elderly people as well as benefiting patients suffering from Alzheimer's disease, myasthenia gravis and Friedrich's ataxia.

lipoic acid

$C_8S_2H_{14}O_2$

This chemical was formerly classified as a B complex vitamin. It is required for the growth of a number of microorganisms species, but it is synthesized in sufficient quantities in the human body so that no intake from the diet is required. The structure is of a fatty acid chain joined by a disulphide bridge. Its function is to help carry out enzyme reactions that catalyse the removal of carbon dioxide groups from certain compounds in the Krebs cycle. This allows the maximum energy to be obtained from each molecule of glucose eaten.

Macrominerals

more than 100mg daily requirement

calcium

chemical symbol: Ca

Calcium is a metal that is widely distributed in nature as carbonate, sulphate, silicate and halide salts. It is found in milk, dairy products, hard tap water, fish (especially sardines and pilchards), white flour, bread, green leafy vegetables and fortified cereals. The mineral is absorbed into our bodies through the intestinal walls, and this process is facilitated by the presence of vitamin D. It is also influenced by the presence of stomach acids and by the intake of dietary fibre and proteins. Calcium also allows uptake of vitamin B_{12} (cyanocobalamin) from the intestines. The recommended dietary allowance for calcium varies between 500mg and 1000mg for healthy adults, with pregnant women requiring 1200mg and women over forty-five being encouraged to take 1500mg per day. There is a wide variety of recommended intake, and some sources state that pregnant women do not need higher levels of calcium as a woman's body absorbs many nutrients better while pregnant. The higher doses recommended for older women are to try to prevent osteoporosis, which is most common in post-menopausal women.

The human body contains large quantities of calcium—generally around 1200g, of which 99 per cent is found in the bones and teeth. Adequate levels of calcium are critical for babies and children while their teeth and bones are growing. Calcium is needed for the transmission of nerve impulses, maintaining the fluid balance and for muscle contraction. It is also important in the coagulation of blood, for cardiac activity and for the secretion of breast milk. Calcium is contained in soft tissue cells and in extracellular fluid where, if levels become elevated, it can trigger muscle weakness, lethargy and even coma. Even small deviations from the normal mineral concentration can cause influx of calcium into the cells, leading to cell damage or death, and prompting seizures. Calcium levels in the blood are generally $100mg/l^{-1}$ and are controlled by a combination of two hormones—thyrocalcitonin, which lowers the levels of calcium and phosphorus in the blood, and parathyroid hormone, which controls the distribution of calcium in the body between the blood and the bones. The amount of calcium in the bones and teeth is not static. There is actually a dynamic system in which

275

calcium is taken away from the bone and replaced each day, showing that skeletal bone is a living tissue with an active metabolism. Any excess calcium may be deposited in the body as calculi, particularly in the kidney or bladder, as tartar on the teeth, or it is excreted via urine, faeces or sweat.

Deficiencies of calcium are rare but can occur because of a lack of vitamin D or a problem with calcium absorption in the intestines. Conditions caused by such a deficiency include rickets in children, with weakened development of bone mass and teeth. The adult form of rickets is called osteomalacia. Rickets in early life may predispose someone to develop osteoporosis in later life. Problems with the levels of calcium in the blood serum can develop because of a tumour affecting the parathyroid glands. Too little calcium intake weakens the bones, teeth, hair and nails and may also lead to allergic reactions developing. Calcium competes with magnesium in the body, and they need to be present in the correct proportions for both to function correctly. Magnesium can reduce high blood levels of calcium, but calcium can also help solve potassium deficiencies. Thus, many of the minerals and trace elements required are interdependent upon the presence of others. Therapeutic supplements of both calcium and magnesium have been used to treat joint problems and are also helpful for osteoporosis. This is the most difficult condition of calcium disorders to treat, and attempts have been made to relieve the disease using combinations of calcium, oestrogen, fluorine, magnesium, silicon and sex hormones. Injections of thyrocalcitonin have proved of some benefit, while fluorine is included to encourage bone growth and reduce the chance of fractures. Results have been mixed, but it has been discovered that calcium requires the presence of both magnesium and silicon for assimilation into the bones. For osteoporosis, prevention is better than cure, and the aim now is to ensure adequate intake of calcium in young women and teenagers as this may be the critical period that decides a person's susceptibility to the disease.

chlorine

chemical symbol: Cl

Chlorine is a trace element that is essential to the formation of digestive stomach acids, e.g. hydrochloric acid, HCl. It is also required for the correct functioning of the carbon dioxide transport system in the blood. When CO_2 bound by the red blood cells reaches the lungs, it can only be released and expelled out of the lungs if the procedure is triggered by the movement of chloride ions through a transmembrane protein found in red blood cells. The transmembrane protein is called the Band III protein, and it is found in the red blood cells of humans, rabbits, rats, salmon and trout, among other species. Chlorine is also very closely linked to sodium, and these elements regulate the acid-base balance, the fluid balance and the osmotic pressure in the blood. In excess of 100mg of chlorine is required per day, but there is generally too much chlorine in our diets in the form of table salt. The human body contains around 75g of chlorine, 60g of which is found in the blood plasma and tissue fluids.

magnesium
chemical symbol: Mg

Like calcium, magnesium is a metallic element that is found in the intracellular fluids of the body. Around 20–28g of magnesium is contained in the human body of an adult, 99 per cent of which is held within the cells. Most of that magnesium is in the bones or muscles, while only 1 per cent is found in the intracellular fluid or blood serum. This explains why analysis of blood serum does not give representative measurement for magnesium levels in the tissues. The RDA for this mineral is around 300mg, with pregnant women and nursing mothers requiring 450mg per day. Good sources of magnesium include green vegetables, wholemeal flour, milk, eggs, fish, pulses, shellfish, nuts (especially peanuts), meat, and cereals and their products. Absorption of the mineral into the bloodstream occurs via the intestines, and this uptake is highly variable. Generally around 30–40 per cent of the magnesium available is taken up, and when less magnesium is available, the percentage absorption increases. Absorption is deleteriously affected by dietary intake of calcium, phosphorus, proteins, saturated animal fat and fibre. The balance of magnesium in humans relates to the level of magnesium in the urine, and this is normally between 100 and 150mg per day. Higher levels of magnesium in the blood serum correlate to an increase in the level of magnesium eliminated via the urine. This process appears to be linked to calcium and sodium loss in the urine. In the body, magnesium is essential for the production and activation of many enzymes that regulate the metabolism of proteins, carbohydrates, lipids, nucleic acids and nucleotides (see Krebs cycle in the Glossary). Magnesium acts as a co-factor for approximately 90 enzymes in energy metabolism.

It is required to allow proper functioning of neurochemical transmissions and is vital for normal muscle function. In the cell it is vital for cell division and for all reactions with phosphates. If cells are deficient in magnesium, the permeability of the cell membranes changes, causing potassium and magnesium to be lost and replaced by sodium and calcium. This ultimately gives rise to a substance called AMP (adenosine monophosphate) that eventually leads to cell death. Magnesium is also needed for healthy bones and teeth and proper nerve function, and it allows vitamins B (thiamin) and B_{12} (cyanocobalamin) to carry out their proper roles in the body. Magnesium acts on the heart muscle and the whole circulatory system as it prevents an increase in blood pressure.

277

Counting Calories

A deficiency of magnesium seems to lead to muscle weakness and fatigue and possible development of cardiac arrhythmia. A lack of the mineral is often see in heart patients and also increases the sensitivity of the heart to digoxin, a common cardiac remedy. Too little magnesium may cause nephrocalcinosis, where calcium deposits form in the kidney tissue, and this can be prevented by magnesium supplementation. Additional magnesium can also reduce the risk of occurrence of myocardial infarction, where a coronary artery becomes blocked, and it also reduces the chances of a second infarction occurring later in life. Around the turn of the century, the daily intake was around 1200mg (between three and four times today's RDA). A study of postmortems carried out at that time showed that out of 1000 individuals, none had died from a heart infarction.

This mineral also plays a role in both the cell and antibody-mediated immune response. If the diets of experimental animals are lacking in magnesium, then the levels of immunoglobulin antibodies is reduced by up to 60 per cent. The effect is especially strong for IgG, but the levels of IgA, IgE and IgM also fall. This process may occur because B-lymphocytes cannot develop into the antibody-producing plasma cells, and magnesium is suggested to be involved in that process in some manner. Further research is being carried out to determine the immunological properties of magnesium. The cell-mediated response consists of T-lymphocytes that require magnesium and calcium for proper maturation. Studies on rats have proved a direct link between magnesium deficiencies and impaired immune defence against allergic reactions and cancers, particularly lymphoma and leukaemia. Up to this point, no large human population studies have been carried out to consider a possible link between magnesium deficiency and disorders of the immune system. Magnesium deficiency in humans can occur because of a low dietary intake, problems with magnesium absorption in the intestines or because of excessive elimination of magnesium in the urine. Certain diseases can increase the level of magnesium lost, e.g. diabetes, kidney diseases and some hormonal disorders. Some drugs, such as diuretic medicines, and alcohol can increase the level of magnesium lost in the urine. A deficiency of magnesium is often accompanied with a lack of potassium, but this may not be easily detected by measuring blood serum only. Measurement of magnesium in the body via the blood cells, platelets or whole blood is far more accurate, but the best results are obtained by measuring magnesium loss through the urine over a 24-hour period. Magnesium deficiency can arise gradually over time, leading to symptoms of anxiety, fatigue, loss of appetite, hormonal disorders, nausea, insomnia, hypoglycaemia, muscle weakness and muscle cramps, and trembling ('restless legs'). A reduced level of magnesium in the body may also be linked to premenstrual tension. A serious deficiency of magnesium can, as mentioned before, lead to arrhythmia, which can be detected on an electrocardiogram (ECG).

This link between magnesium and heart problems has been studied since the 1960s, when it was found that there is a reduced incidence of heart disease in areas with hard water. Hard water contains calcium and magnesium, and this may supplement the dietary supply of these minerals. Thus, supplementation of the diet with magnesium may benefit a range of heart problems. This process does not harm the body, has a low cost and yet can reduce the damage after heart infarction and decreases the risk of fatal cardiac arrhythmia. Investigations in Denmark and Finland have shown that magnesium deficiency in the blood exists prior to a heart attack, and supplement therapy can reduce the risk of a repeated attack. Magnesium deficiency is also seen in cases of allergy or asthma that have been successfully treated with supplements. The mineral supplements seem to reduce the levels of histamine in the blood and allow the patient's condition to improve. Magnesium has an antihistamine effect and can alleviate the symptoms of many asthmatic patients or those with atopic eczema. Magnesium also is a mild tranquillizer and can replace tranquillizing medicines to some degree. Finally, the physical and psychological symptoms associated with undefined fatigue can be treated successfully with magnesium supplement.

Recent work has found a possible connection between breast cancer and blood levels of magnesium. This has yet to be substantiated, but it may be probable that low magnesium levels can predispose a person to developing cancer. At a conference in the United States, evidence was shown of correlations between insufficient magnesium intake and the onset of high blood pressure, cardiovascular diseases and complications in pregnancy. Many research workers now believe that 80 per cent of the United States population gets less than the recommended dietary intake of magnesium. Those most at risk are people who take diuretic or antibiotic drugs or heart medicines, which interfere with the normal metabolism of magnesium, and people who consume excessive amounts of alcohol. Some reports state that magnesium deficiency during pregnancy could result in migraines and in pregnancy-related high blood pressure. Miscarriage, stillbirths and low-birth-weight babies may be linked to inadequate supplies of magnesium. In animal experiments, supplementation with magnesium was said to reduce high blood pressure and limit the impact of arteriosclerosis in animals on a high cholesterol diet. Whether such actions can translate to humans remains to be seen.

phosphorus
chemical symbol: P
This is a nonmetallic element that is found in nature as phosphate salts. It is found in nearly all foodstuffs but particularly in high protein foods

---

such as meat, dairy products, pulses and milk as well as most fruits and leafy green vegetables. The RDA for the mineral is 800mg for healthy adults and 1200mg for pregnant women and nursing mothers. Lack of phosphorus can cause weight loss, demineralization of bone, weakness, loss of appetite and stiff joints. Other problems of phosphorus deficiency include anaemia, central nerve disorders and respiratory failure. A deficiency of phosphorus can affect bone density as it is required to form calcium phosphate, one of the main components of bone tissue. At the other extreme, too much phosphorus in the diet can interfere with absorption of calcium, iron, magnesium and zinc from the intestines.

Phosphorus is essential for many enzymes involved in glucose, protein and fat metabolism, e.g. phosphoglycerokinase in glycolysis. Phosphate also plays a part in adenosine triphosphate (ATP), which is vital throughout the energy production process, and in energy storage in humans. The majority of phosphorus is contained in the bones and teeth. Phosphorus is also essential to the formation of nucleic acids used in cell division.

potassium

chemical symbol: K

This is a metallic element that is required for the correct functioning of all plants and animals. It is found in most foods, including fresh fruits, vegetables (particularly potatoes), meat, milk, wholemeal flour, coffee, tea, cereals and their products, and salt substitutes. On average, a diet of 2800kcal contains 3–4g of potassium, and most people consume 2–4g per day. Somewhat surprisingly, around 15 per cent of our intake comes from coffee, which contains about 45mg of potassium per cup. The human body contains approximately 115–150g of the mineral, 98 per cent of which is held inside the cells. Potassium has an important role in the nervous system, the heart and the muscles. Its role is closely linked to that of sodium, as they have opposite effects. Potassium ions are the main alkaline ions found in the intracellular fluid and, along with sodium, it controls and maintains the electrical potential of the nervous system, which allows the transmission of nerve impulses out through the body. It helps regulate muscle contraction and neuromuscular excitability. Potassium also acts to maintain the body's osmotic balance and is also required by the heart muscle. A correct balance of potassium is needed to prevent arrhythmia. The mineral is also involved in several enzyme systems and in the metabolism of protein. Potassium uptake from the blood into the cells is possible only if magnesium is present, so supplementation of both minerals may be required to prevent any deficiency. Normal levels of potassium in the blood are between 3.5 and 5mmol/litre.

Potassium in the diet does not pose any risks to health in the same way that sodium does. Like many other minerals, potassium is absorbed through the intestines, and any excess is eliminated in the urine. If the intake is less than the level excreted, then potassium levels in the cells and blood serum will decrease. To replace these K+ ions, the cells use H+ ions or protons, which can cause problems by changing the cells' acidity. Increased loss of potassium in the urine can occur because of increased intake of alcohol, coffee and sugar. Diuretic drugs also increase the levels of potassium and magnesium lost, so treatment with these medicines should always be followed by checks of the potassium balance of the patient. Some diuretic drugs try to overcome this problem by retaining potassium in the body or by containing potassium themselves to supplement the intake. Symptoms of this mineral deficiency include muscle weakness, fatigue, fluid accumulation, 'pins and needles', loss of appetite, thirst, constipation, low blood pressure, and disorders of the kidneys and nervous systems. Inadequate potassium levels also affect the heart and change the way it is affected by some drugs, e.g. digitalis. It can lead to a higher risk of digitalis poisoning. Paralysis may result from insufficient potassium as the nerve impulses cannot be generated properly. Conversely, high levels of potassium in the blood can occur because of excessive fluid loss caused by prolonged vomiting or diarrhoea, producing symptoms of drowsiness, sensations of disorientation, weakness and cardiac problems including arrhythmia. This may finally lead to cardiac arrest. Excess potassium may occur because of kidney failure as the mineral cannot be eliminated effectively, and this can be shown on an electrocardiogram (ECG). Very high levels of potassium intake can reduce the effectiveness of anticoagulant medicines, and the dosage of such drugs may need to be raised during the summer when consumption of potassium-containing vegetables rises. Levels of potassium in the blood may be upset and reduced by diseases of the heart, liver and kidney, as well as by diabetes, cancer and hyperthyrosis, which is a hyperactive thyroid gland. Both too little and too much potassium can lead to metabolic disturbances.

Potassium supplements can be used to remedy several problems. Deficiency of the mineral because of diuretic drugs can be treated by giving a preventative dose of 1–2g daily or by administering 2–4g supplements per day, after checking the blood levels for potassium. This mineral may help reduce the accumulation of fluid in the body tissues, but this may not be advised during pregnancy. The source of the fluid retention should first be investigated before any treatment is given. In most cases where the swelling poses no threat to health, then potassium therapy may be safer than the use of diuretic drugs, which may deplete the body of minerals and vitamins. The excessive intake of coffee has diuretic properties and may cause deficiency in potassium despite the fact that coffee is a rich source of the mineral. Potassium tablets can cause problems as they may trigger stomach trouble or constipation, or irritate the mucous membranes. In susceptible people, such tablets may even trigger the development of a duodenal ulcer. They may also stick in the oesophagus unless taken with plenty of water. Some tablets are formulated to be slow-releasing, and they cause fewer side effects than the other tablets. Potassium supplementation is not tolerated well by patients with kidney failure.

Both potassium and magnesium deficiencies produce symptoms that are similar, and insufficient levels of one implies the other is also lacking. As mentioned before, both potassium and magnesium are required for uptake of potassium in the cells. If not, the blood serum values for potassium increases but not the cellular values. Calcium can correct symptoms caused by potassium deficiency but only to a certain extent.

sodium

chemical symbol: Na

Like potassium, sodium is a metal whose ions are the chief electrolyte in intracellular fluid. There is around 100g of sodium in the body, of which 50 per cent is found in the cells, primarily the bone cells. It is a major essential element for most animals, and humans require around 3g per day. We ingest sodium as sodium chloride, and it is added to many tinned, cured or processed foods, including cured meats, milk, smoked fish, bakery products, and tinned meat and vegetables. Most people use table salt, and as a consequence many people consume far too much salt, between 5 and 15g per day, or up to five times the recommended level. Around 50 per cent of our salt intake comes from preprocessed food, and 40 per cent is added at the table. Only 12 per cent of our intake actually comes from the sodium contained naturally in our food. Sodium may also be taken in by soft drinks, sodium-rich mineral waters or by headache tablets that contain acetyl salicylate (aspirin).

Sodium is critical to many processes in the body. Sodium ions are the main ions in intracellular fluid, and their interaction with potassium ions across cell membranes is required for survival. This process maintains the electrical potentials in the nervous system and permits normal functioning of nerves and muscles. The mineral is also involved with sustaining the acid-alkali balance, the production of adrenaline and the manufacturing of amino acids. Sodium also controls the water balance in the body.

The uptake of sodium from the small intestine and the stomach is easy, and the mineral goes on to be filtered from the bloodstream by the kidneys. Generally, over 90 per cent of sodium intake is eliminated from the body along with the urine. The main problem is excessive salt intake, which can raise blood pressure in people susceptible to this condition. High sodium levels can also aggravate or sustain already high blood pressure, and it may contribute to migraine attacks. It may also lead to a condition called hypernatraemia, which can cause fluid retention (oedema), mental confusion, seizures, and even coma. It can be treated by restoring the electrolyte balance in the body and may occur in bottle-fed babies as artificial milk has a much higher sodium content than breast milk. The babies cannot remove sodium from the body as efficiently as adults so dehydration may occur.

A deficiency of sodium is rare, but it may occur if sodium recycling is affected by a kidney malfunction. Sodium deficiency may arise if there is heavy sweat secretion because of a high workload or hot conditions. Symptoms of insufficient sodium include low blood pressure, weakness in the muscles, mild fever, respiratory problems, dizziness, loss of weight and general indisposition.

One of the prime reasons for hypertension, heart disorders and kidney complaints is excessive salt intake. Healthy salt habits should be taught in childhood as it becomes increasingly difficult to break our salt habits as we get older. Reduced intake of sodium may reduce our chances of developing high blood pressure in later life. We can replace sodium by the use of herbs, spices and herbal salt as seasonings and by using a salt substitute such as Pan-Salt or Lo-Salt, where some of the sodium chloride is replaced with potassium chloride to reduce our intake of sodium.

sulphur

chemical symbol: S

This is a yellow nonmetallic element that is required to form part of the amino acids cysteine and methionine. It is found in animal and vegetable proteins contained in meat, dairy products, pulses and nuts. There is no official RDA for this element, but it is essential for the formation of many proteins to make skin, nails and strong hair. Sulphur is also required for the proper development of cartilage and tendons, and it makes up part of many cell metabolites, such as co-enzyme A. Deficiency of sulphur is very rare and would occur only if there were insufficient intake of proteins that lack the amino acids that contain sulphur.

Microminerals

Fewer than 1mg–100mg daily requirement

bromine

chemical symbol: Br

Bromine would not seem to be required by the human body, although we take in between 1.5 and 2.5mg per day through our diets. Bromide salts of sodium, potassium and strontium are used in medicine as sedatives, hypnotics and analgesics. Their use dates back to the late 1880s, and bromides were formerly the standard treatment for epilepsy as they depress the activity of the central nervous system. They have largely been replaced by more recent anticonvulsant drugs but are still used occasionally in cases that will not respond to the new treatments. Bromides may be given in cases of insomnia, but the drug may produce a particular form of acne to erupt. Long-term use of bromides can lead to mental dullness, drowsiness, weakness, slurred speech, loss of sensation, and even coma. The problems can be rectified by immediate withdrawal of the drug.

chromium

chemical symbol: Cr

Chromium is a metallic element that is essential for normal body function. The amount of chromium required for health is unsure, but American authorities estimate that between 50 and 200μg is a safe and adequate dose. Chromium exists in an organic and inorganic form, with around 25 per cent of organic chromium being absorbed into the body against only 0.5 per cent of the inorganic form. Chromium is found in meat, unrefined and unprocessed foods, particularly wholemeal flour, cereals and cereal products, cheese, nuts, liver, brewer's yeast, fresh fruits, and herbs. Like most minerals, chromium is absorbed through the intestines and taken into the blood where it is bound by a protein called transferrin. After a period of time, chromium is released from the blood and stored in the liver, bone marrow and the spleen. In these tissues, chromium is found in association with vitamin B_3 (niacin). Absorption of chromium is inhibited by iron, manganese, zinc, titanium and calcium. Any excess of chromium is eliminated via the urine, and only a minute quantity is lost via the sweat or faeces. Like potassium and magnesium, the level of chromium in the blood serum or whole blood is tiny and does not reflect the chromium balance in the body. The only way to assess accurately the chromium balance is to measure the amounts of chromium excreted in the urine.

Chromium's role in the human body is not entirely clear, but it does seem to play a part in the functioning of skeletal muscles, helps in controlling the immune system and is involved in the metabolism and storage of sugars and fats. Animal studies have shown that lack of chromium causes reduced protein production, shorter life-span, eye damage and lowered fertility. Insufficient chromium in rats and monkeys has led to a decreased glucose tolerance, which can be resolved with supplements of the mineral. This link to glucose would also seem to occur in humans, and it has been suggested that chromium is part of the glucose tolerance factor molecule (GTF). This molecule is responsible for the foundation of a balance in sugar metabolism, but it has not yet been isolated. Recent studies have led doctors to believe that chromium is able to prevent hypoglycaemia, or low blood sugar levels. Conflicting results about this possibility have arisen, largely because of a lack of adequate control groups and variability in the preparations and dosage of chromium used.

Chromium deficiency may cause weakness, confusion, irritability and depression. It may also be a contributory factor in arteriosclerosis, as postmortem findings have shown that people with arteriosclerosis have very low values of chromium. Chromium values fall with advancing age in countries with higher levels of arteriosclerosis, in contrast to countries with little or no arteriosclerosis problem. Arteriosclerosis and heart disease are a particular problem in eastern Finland, for example, where the average daily intake of chromium is approximately $30\mu g$ and there are deficiencies in selenium also.

Some studies have proposed that organic chromium may be able to reduce the levels of fat in the blood. Further research is needed to shed some light on this possibility. Currently, chromium has no scientific basis for use as a therapy. Some nutritional doctors have prescribed chromium, either alone or with zinc and selenium, as therapy for people with coronary artery disease, diabetes, arrhythmia and hypoglycaemia. Several studies in Finland and Korea have shown that chromium supplements in diabetic patients can reduce the sugar levels in their blood, leading to less insulin requirement. Many patients have fewer symptoms and improved general health, and some people were able to stop taking insulin altogether. For chromium to regulate the sugar balance effectively requires a small quantity of insulin in the blood, so it works only in people who had a functioning pancreas, even if only to a small degree. The beneficial effects were also stopped if medicines that counteracted chromium were being taken. Chromium can also help patients with symptomatic hypoglycaemia, which causes headaches, anxiety,

Counting Calories

visual disturbances and general discomfort. Chromium is one of the minerals that warrants further study into its role in the human body.

cobalt

chemical symbol: Co

Cobalt is an essential trace element that forms part of the molecule of vitamin B_{12} (cyanocobalamin). It is found in meat, milk, eggs, green vegetables, figs and buckwheat. The human body contains about 1mg of cobalt, on average, and this is found in the muscles and bones. The role of cobalt in the body is as an essential component of vitamin B_{12}, and also it appears to stimulate the production of a glycoprotein hormone, called erythropoietin, when there is a lack of oxygen in the body. The reason for this action is unknown. Cobalt is taken into the body through the small intestines, and humans can tolerate quite large quantities of the mineral, side effects only arising if the daily intake is more than 20–30mg. The side effects can include a weakening of heart functioning and thyroid failure. There is no set RDA for this mineral as its role in humans is poorly understood. Deficiency of cobalt would result in insufficient vitamin B_{12}, which leads to weak muscles, bowel and nerve disorders, and pernicious anaemia. Some use of cobalt as a therapy in various types of anaemia has been attempted, as it has for reducing high blood pressure, but its use as a treatment has never been accepted.

An isotope of cobalt, Cobalt 60, is radioactive and has been used successfully to treat cancer with penetrating gamma-radiation.

copper

chemical symbol: Cu

Copper is an essential mineral that fulfils many roles in the body. There is about 80mg of copper inside the average human, most of it in the liver, brain, muscles, heart and the bones. The RDA for copper is between 2 and 5mg per day, and this comes from shellfish (particularly oysters), cocoa, tap water, liver, kidney, raisins, peas, nuts (particularly brazil nuts) and brewer's yeast. Copper is absorbed in both the stomach and the small intestine, and if the body reserves are full, then excess copper is excreted in the faeces and absorption drops by 80–90 per cent. Absorption is also affected by the presence of fibre or protein in the intestine as well as cadmium, iron, zinc, cobalt and molybdenum. Copper is particularly affected by zinc as the two minerals compete to form compounds with proteins. In the blood, copper is found in the red blood cells and the plasma. In the red blood cells, some of the copper is loosely attached to amino acids, and this reserve is called the labile pool or metabolic storage. Most of the copper in the red blood cells (60 per cent) is bound to the enzyme copper-zinc superoxide dismutase (CuZn SOD), which is called the stable pool or permanent storage. Currently,

286

little is known about the copper metabolism or the movement of the copper reserves from pool to pool. This CuZn SOD enzyme contains two copper and two zinc atoms, and it protects the cells from free radicals and peroxides, especially superoxides that have a structure of O_2- and are produced in respiration.

The copper held in the plasma is usually bound to a protein called ceruloplasmin. This protein is dark blue in colour, is produced in the liver and contains eight copper atoms. It acts as a natural antioxidant and is found in elevated levels during infection or inflammation when the body is exposed to excess free radicals. Ceruloplasmin also regulates the level of the hormones melatonin, adrenaline, noradrenaline and serotonin in the blood plasma. The protein is needed for the production of red blood cells as it stops storage of iron in the liver and directs it to the blood cells. Deficiency of copper, and so ceruloplasmin, causes easier oxidation of iron, and this may contribute to the production of superoxide radicals in cells. The levels of ceruloplasmin in the blood rise during physical activity.

The levels of copper in the blood are normally $90–145\mu gl^{-1}$ in plasma and $85–125\mu gl^{-1}$ in whole blood. This can change because of oestrogen treatment and pregnancy. Copper values rise during infection (because of the increased amounts of ceruloplasmin in the blood), and this can be used to gauge the activity of diseases such as arthritis.

As mentioned previously, copper has an active role in the superoxide dismutase (SOD) enzyme. The CuZn SOD enzyme is the fifth most common protein in the human organism and is found in the red blood cells and all tissues. Its job is to make oxygen-free radicals harmless to the cells in a similar way to the selenium enzyme glutathione peroxidase. Tests have been done to see if this enzyme can be used as a therapy for some diseases, e.g. inflamed joints in arthritis. Results showed a short-lasting but beneficial effect, and it was found that SOD was more effective in reducing the level of the rheumatoid factor than aspirin-type drugs. SOD was also seen to reduce the levels of PGE2, which is a harmful prostaglandin chemical. SOD has proved effective in easing osteoarthritis as well, and more studies should reveal the range of conditions this enzyme may help.

Another enzyme that requires copper is cytochrome oxidase, and it is absolutely critical for the metabolism. If copper is deficient then levels of the enzyme fall and energy production in the cells falls also. This has a large knock-on effect on the whole food metabolism of the body. Copper is found in two other enzymes—ascorbic acid oxidase and tyrosinases.

Copper deficiency is fairly rare but can result in serious diseases such as Menke's syndrome or Wilson's disease. Deficiency can result from problems with the absorption of food because of a biliary obstruction or an inflamed liver caused by biliary cirrhosis. Symptoms of insufficient copper include hair loss, changes in hair colour and texture, diarrhoea, anaemia, disturbances to the nervous system, low white blood cell count, and bone diseases. Inadequate copper intake in children can lead to brittle bones and inhibition of growth. Lack of copper can lead to an elevated risk of heart and circulatory complaints, particularly if it occurs with a deficiency of selenium. This would affect the activity of both major antioxidant enzymes, CuZn SOD and glutathione peroxidase, allowing free radicals to do much more cell damage. This problem is particularly bad for people with constricted blood vessels because oxygen deficiency (ischaemia) encourages the production of free radicals.

At the onset of an infection of any origin, the levels of ceruloplasmin and copper in the blood serum rise within a few hours. Amounts of zinc in the blood fall quickly at the same time as the copper levels rise when a person has an infectious disease such as tuberculosis of the lung. This means values of zinc and copper in the blood can be used as an indirect guide to hidden infections in some part of the body. In most cases, the levels of both minerals in the blood return to normal after a few weeks.

Copper levels in the blood are also affected by malignant tumours in the body. Cancers of the womb, lungs, breast and bladder cause increased copper in the blood, as does Hodgkin's disease and non-Hodgkin's lymphoma. Cancer of the prostate shows no changes in blood levels of copper. So elevated blood levels of the mineral should be investigated further, but they do not automatically mean that cancer is present in the body. Medicinal treatment of cancer returns copper levels to normal, and any rise in level thereafter may indicate a possible relapse of the disease.

fluorine

chemical symbol: F

Elemental fluorine exists as a gas, but it is used in the human body as fluoride salts. There is between 3 and 7mg of fluorine in the average adult and that normally comes from fluoridated drinking water, toothpastes, tea, cereals, meat and fish (especially sardines, herring and mackerel). The American RDA is from 1.0 to 4.0mg daily for healthy adults. Dietary fluoride is quickly and totally absorbed into the body, and fats can increase the level of absorption. Absorption is reduced by calcium, sodium chloride and aluminium. The fluoride is moved to the bones, teeth, kidneys, the aorta and other tissues via the blood. Levels of fluorine in soft tissues stay relatively constant over time, but levels in the bones increase with age. Excess fluoride is excreted in the urine, and it reflects both the level of intake and the previous intake of the mineral. Kidney complaints change or stop the level of fluorine loss.

The main role of fluoride is to be incorporated into tooth enamel, making the teeth more resistant to dental caries and attack by bacteria and plaque acids. Fluoride ions enter enamel as it is forming and also after teeth have erupted by absorption through the surfaces. There is some debate as to whether the addition of fluoride to the water is acceptable. Much of the evidence shows that water containing up to 1 part per million of fluoride results in reduced incidence of dental caries. Fluoridation of water would appear to be the easiest way to ensure the majority of the population receives enough fluoride. There is also some debate as to whether fluoride can strengthen the bones and prevent or slow down osteoporosis. Conflicting results have been found in studies from France, Finland and Denmark, where people were treated with fluoride to help osteoporosis. One of the Finnish studies thought that additional fluoride may increase the risk of breaking the femora or thigh bone. It has been agreed that fluorine, along with calcium and vitamin D, can increase the bone mass in osteoporotic patients. The new bone mass hardens but the tissue formed does not compare to normal bone composition.

Fluoride may have some link with the incidence of cardiovascular disease. Several studies have shown both an increased and decreased risk with fluoride intake, and these ambiguous results may be because of the variation in methods of study or external factors such as dietary habits, vitamin and mineral intake, the hardness of the water and the level of pollutants in the environment. Excessive intake of fluoride can cause problems, including fluorosis, a condition that results in discoloration and mottling of the teeth. Other problems may include calcification of the ligaments and increased density of the bones of the spine, pelvis and limbs.

Fluoride deficiency is uncommon in humans, but in animals it can cause limited growth, disorders in the development of teeth, and hair loss.

iodine

chemical symbol: I

Similar to fluorine, iodine is a gas in its simplest form but commonly forms iodide salts. The human body contains only 20–50μg of iodine, but it plays a critical role in the production of many hormones, and it is linked to proper growth and development. Iodine is found in iodized table salt, seafood including seaweed, meat, and fruit and vegetables in areas where the soil contains iodine. The average adult needs 100–200μg of iodine daily, and deficiencies can cause serious problems. Almost 80 per cent of the iodine found in the body is in the thyroid gland, where iodine is bound to the amino acid tyrosine. Iodine is used to produce the thyroid hormones thyroxine (T4) and triiodothyronine (T3). These hormones act to increase the metabolic rate, regulate carbohydrate, protein and fat catabolism, promote development of the central nervous system, and stimulate the synthesis of many other enzymes. They also sustain secretion of growth hormone, are necessary for muscle tone and vigour, and maintain the heart rate, its force and its output, as well as ensuring proper skeletal maturation. For a small gland, it plays a large role in development through childhood and then continuing through our adult lives. Iodine's role in the thyroid gland was first noticed in 1818. Dietary iodine is absorbed, and a third of it goes directly to the thyroid gland while the rest is eliminated in the urine. Unusually, the iodine that is lost also seems to have some effect on our bodies before elimination but what happens precisely is not yet known.

Deficiency of iodine can result in a drop in the metabolic rate, which causes fatigue, drowsiness, lethargy and weight gain. Reduced production of the thyroid hormones in pregnancy or in the early life of an infant can cause a disease called cretinism. The child suffers from dwarfism, mental retardation, and coarse facial features and skin. If the condition is detected early enough (within the first six weeks of life) then treatment with injections of thyroid hormones can significantly help the condition. Several countries have set up automatic biochemical screening programmes in order to trace cases of cretinism early.

The main problem of iodine deficiency is a disease called goitre. It occurs in four forms, but all result in swelling of the neck caused by enlargement of the thyroid gland. This occurs because of a lack of dietary iodine so the gland grows in order to produce more hormone (endemic goitre), because of simple excessive growth of the gland (sporadic goitre), or because of overactivity of the gland, sometimes caused by autoimmune diseases, such as in lymphadenoid goitre or Grave's disease (exothalmic goitre). Iodine deficiency was common in parts of Europe up to the 1940s and 1950s. Then iodine was added to table salt, increasing the dietary intake of iodine, and the problem was solved. Iodine deficiency still occurs in some areas of Africa, South America and Asia. Iodine tablets have been used to reduce the dangers of radioactive radiation in people who have been exposed to excessive radiation, e.g. people exposed to fallout or radiation from the Chernobyl disaster or some workers in the nuclear industry. Iodine isotopes that emit radioactivity are used in scanning procedures, e.g. of the gall bladder, and in treatment of some cancers. Iodine is widely used as a skin disinfectant.

iron

chemical symbol: Fe
Iron is a metallic element essential to life and many biological processes. The average adult has around 4g of iron in the body, 65 per cent

in haemoglobin, 10 per cent in the myoglobin, while the rest is stored in the liver, kidneys, spleen, the bone marrow and other organs. The RDA for adults is 14–18mg and 30–60mg in pregnant women. Iron supplementation is given as the rule to breast-feeding women as well. Iron occurs in three forms, haem iron from meat, non-haem iron from vegetables, and non-haem iron added to foodstuffs. Each type is absorbed with differing degrees of difficulty, and absorption of any iron from the diet is generally poor, at around 5 per cent of the dietary intake. The best sources of iron are meat (especially liver), offal, blood, peas, parsley, pulses, eggs, whole grains, green leafy vegetables, nuts (particularly almonds), cocoa, apricots and figs, fortified white flour and products, and fortified breakfast cereals. In meat, 40 per cent of the meat is haem iron, and generally around 24 per cent of this is absorbed. This figure may seem low but actually reflects a good level of absorption. Haem-iron uptake is not affected by other dietary components. Non-haem iron is more difficult in uptake and generally is significantly affected by other substances in the diet. Coffee, tea and calcium all inhibit the absorption of iron, but it is increased by vitamin C. The calcium in milk, for example, competes with iron and makes it less available for uptake into the bloodstream. Wheat flour and some breakfast cereals are commonly fortified with iron. At first glance this may seem beneficial, but there is a range of formulations of iron that are added to the foodstuffs. Most countries add iron as ferrous iron powder that is absorbed pretty well without any interference from other foods. In Sweden, iron is added as ferric orthosulphate, which is taken up by the body particularly well. A problem may arise with the soluble ferrosulphate that is added to breast-milk substitutes, as it tends to react with the fats in the milk, leading to lipid peroxidation.

Iron is absorbed into the body through the upper section of the small intestine, changing from ferrous to ferric iron in the process. It then enters the blood, where most of the iron binds to the protein called transferrin. Some iron remains in the free state in the blood serum. The mineral then binds itself to the protein haemoglobin in the red blood cells. This procedure requires vitamin E, copper, cobalt and molybdenum to be present. Haemoglobin is the respiratory pigment found in the blood of all vertebrates, and it is composed of the haem group, composed of iron and porphyrin, a natural pigment, and the protein globin. Haemoglobin exists in two forms—oxyhaemoglobin, which is formed in the lungs and carries oxygen to all the body tissues, where it is reduced and the oxygen is released. This reduced haemoglobin is purplish in colour, compared to the scarlet of oxyhaemoglobin. As well as transporting oxygen, haemoglobin carries carbon dioxide to the lungs, where it is exhaled, and it helps regulate the acidity of the blood. Iron is also moved via the blood to the myoglobin found in the muscles.

Counting Calories

Myoglobin is similar to haemoglobin but smaller in size. It is used for oxygen production in the muscles during periods of oxygen deficiency and acts as an emergency oxygen store. Iron is also found in the cyto-chromes, which are protein-haem compounds important because they act as electron transfer agents in biological reactions. They are found associated with mitochondria inside cells and are very important in the electron transport chain. Iron is stored in an iron-protein complex, called ferritin, and in haemosiderin, which is a protein shell containing iron salts, both of which are stored in the tissues. As already mentioned, iron is needed for the production of red blood corpuscles and to trans-port oxygen round the body, and it also allows many enzymes to func-tion well. Iron is also required for energy production in the cells. Iron is essential for the metabolism of all the B vitamins.

Deficiency of iron normally results from an unvaried diet, unhealthy eating habits, inadequate intake of vitamin C, and too little meat in the diet. Lack of iron results in anaemia, which is the most common nutri-tional deficiency disease in the industrialized world. Anaemia normally occurs because of a decreased capacity to absorb the mineral, caused by lack of vitamin C or the presence of inhibitory chemicals. Anaemia may be caused by heavy menstrual bleeding and haemorrhaging in the gastrointestinal tract because of cancer, stomach ulcers or haemor-rhoids. Rheumatic complaints and long-term infections can also reduce the body's reserves of iron. Iron loss may be about 0.8–1.0mg per day in adults, but during menstruation women may lose around 1.4mg per day. Anaemia may also be caused by insufficient intake of vitamin B_9 (folic acid) or vitamin B_{12} (cyanocobalamin), which are necessary, along with iron, to form haemoglobin. Symptoms of anaemia include tired-ness, pale skin, breathlessness, loss of strength, nervousness, feeling weak, fainting and palpitations. The haemoglobin content of the blood is normally 12–16g per 100ml, and if this falls below 12g per 100ml, a person is considered anaemic.

Other problems of iron deficiency include a weakening of the white blood cell defence system, which leaves an increased risk of contracting infectious diseases. Iron is also required for the proper functioning of the T-lymphocytes and for enabling them to identify virus, bacteria and cancer cells. Diet supplementation with iron can reduce the number of cases of anaemia and respiratory tract infections in children. Iron sup-plementation can show dramatic effects in formerly deficient people and improves their physical state very rapidly. This is not only because of the increased levels of haemoglobin produced but is possibly linked to a number of actions that iron has in the body, which we do not yet understand completely. Further research is needed into the links be-tween iron deficiency, iron supplementation and infectious diseases to discover the additional properties of iron in the body. There are unusual conditions where excessive amounts of iron can accumulate in the tissues. Haemochromatosis, also called bronze diabetes, occurs because of excessive absorption and storage of iron in the liver, spleen and endocrine glands. Liver failure commonly occurs, as does diabetes mellitus and the development of bronze-pigmented skin. Haemosiderosis is a similar condition in which excessive deposition of iron in the body causes damage to various organs, particularly the liver and the heart. The iron is deposited as haemosiderin, a natural iron storage compound. Polycythaemia occurs because of an increase in the number of red blood cells in the blood. Increased levels of platelets and white blood cells are also seen. This condition occurs naturally at high altitudes as a reaction to the lower oxygen content of air but may also be triggered by heart and lung diseases. The cause of the disease is unknown, and treatment is either by removing some blood cells by blood-letting or using cytotoxic drugs to kill some blood cells. A side effect of very high levels of iron in the body is an increased level of receptivity to infectious diseases.

An iron tablet supplement is normally required for pregnant women and anaemic people. Such problems can cause side effects, including stomach pains, diarrhoea, indisposition and constipation. These problems can be reduced if iron is taken after meals, although this has to be balanced against reduced absorption of the mineral. The dose given may have to be reduced if stomach problems arise. In iron-deficient anaemia, it can take up to six months to correct the iron balance in the body. This can be delayed or even impossible if there is internal bleeding because of a stomach ulcer or if there is severe menstrual bleeding. Once the anaemia is corrected, the supplements should be stopped to reduce the risk of excessive iron reserves in the tissues developing. It is best if two hours pass after taking iron supplements before taking other minerals. This is because iron competes with calcium and manganese in the diet, and these minerals can affect the absorption of iron. The other side of the coin is that long-term iron supplements can lead to insufficient levels of calcium and manganese in the body. Some medicines, such as broad-spectrum antibiotics, should not be taken with iron as the drug forms insoluble compounds with mineral salts.

manganese

chemical symbol: Mn

This metal with antioxidant properties is an essential mineral in our bodies. Manganese is found in nuts, tea, whole-grain cereals, vegetables, pulses and avocados. The RDA is 2.5–3.8mg, and most daily intakes are between 5 and 6mg so there is little occurrence of deficiency. Absorption of the mineral is poor, and only 3 per cent of the manganese in food is absorbed in the organism. Manganese is lost through the urine, and this is increased with alcohol intake. The mineral is stored in the cells, primarily in pigmented cells of the skin, hair and the retina of the eye. The role of manganese in the body is for the formation of strong, healthy bones, for healthy nerves and muscles, and for the control of growth. Manganese forms part of the superoxide dismutase (SOD) enzyme system, and it also helps various enzymes to function effectively. The mineral is important for fertility and in the metabolism of carbohydrates and fats. An inadequate supply of manganese results in a decreased growth rate and bone deformities, but such conditions are uncommon. Deficiencies of manganese produced experimentally have symptoms of reduced hair growth, rashes and other skin changes, and emaciation. Insufficient manganese has been proposed as a contributory factor in epilepsy and diabetes, but further work and studies are required to confirm this hypothesis.

Excess intake of manganese can cause brain damage and symptoms similar to those seen in Parkinson's disease. This has been seen in some miners, who would have inhaled manganese oxide while working in unventilated mine shafts. Conventional medicine does not recognize manganese as a therapy, but some nutritional doctors and alternative medicine practitioners use supplements of the mineral to help patients with painful joints and bones. Since manganese activates the body's killer cells, it may be prescribed in cases of cancer. Supplementation should only occur after blood tests are done to check the levels of mineral in the blood. Care should be taken, as manganese competes with iron so absorption of manganese rises if iron is lacking.

molybdenum

chemical symbol: Mo
This is a metallic element whose role in the human body is largely unknown. It is termed an essential trace element as it forms part of at least three enzymes. Molybdenum is found in buckwheat, barley, oats, liver, leguminous fruits and pulses. The content of molybdenum in foodstuffs varies considerably, depending on the level of the mineral found naturally in the soil. Some areas of Russia have high levels of molybdenum in the soil, and this results in a daily intake of 10–15mg, which is almost one hundred times the normal daily intake. The RDA for this mineral ranges from 100 to 500μg, depending on each country's conditions. Molybdenum is taken into the body and distributed throughout the body tissues, and is found in particularly high levels in the liver. Excess molybdenum is excreted in both the urine and the faeces.

There is little known about what molybdenum does in the body, but it is part of at least three active metabolic enzymes that act to neutralize toxic sulphur compounds. Molybdenum is important in the production of haemoglobin, and it is also supposed to help prevent dental caries.

This effect has been seen in animals and is backed by evidence that levels of dental decay are lower in molybdenum-rich areas. Molybdenum may also be linked to the male sexual function, although this is as yet unproven. In areas where molybdenum content of the soil, and hence of the diet, is extremely low, high levels of cancer of the oesophagus are seen. This may be caused by a failure of the molybdenum enzyme, leading to an accumulation of carcinogenic nitrogen compounds in the tissues. Some animal studies have backed this idea, but the real story is yet to be confirmed. Levels of molybdenum in the blood serum rise above the normal levels of $1.1\mu g$ l^{-1} during liver diseases. Several hereditary diseases result in poor metabolism of molybdenum as two enzymes, xanthine oxidase and sulphite oxidase, do not function well. Molybdenum supplements do not help prevent the illness, and fortunately these diseases are very rare.

Conflicting evidence is available for the importance of this mineral and for its action on the body. Some sources suggest that inadequate intake of molybdenum may lead to increased levels of dental caries, impotence and, in extreme cases, an irregular heartbeat and coma. These deficiency problems may not be true, and molybdenum needs to be researched thoroughly in order to fill in the gaps in our knowledge of it.

selenium

chemical symbol: Se

Selenium is an element that is essential for human health and is found in the same group of the periodic table as oxygen. Selenium was first discovered in 1817 by Jöns J. Berzelius of Sweden. It is found in unrefined foods, especially whole-grain flour, seafood, egg yolk, fish, cereals and products, liver, kidney, garlic and brewer's yeast. The use of selenium as a therapeutic medicine first started around the 1900s when doctors tried to use selenium to treat cancer in France, Britain, Germany and the United States. Unfortunately, the dosages administered were too high, causing selenium poisoning, and much of the medical profession turned against its medicinal use. Through the 1930s, evidence showing selenium poisoning of animals arose in America. This was because of the high levels of selenium in cattle feed, and experiments have confirmed that large doses of selenium can be toxic for animals. Evidence that selenium may be an important nutrient for humans started to arise in 1941, and in 1949 it was proved that selenium could prevent the formation of liver tumours in rats. The first breakthrough occurred in 1957, when Dr Klaus Schwartz discovered that liver necrosis in rats could be prevented by kidney extract, which contained selenium. Since then, selenium has become the focus of a large programme of research.

Early experiments revealed that selenium could prevent muscular dystrophy in pigs, sheep, hens and calves. It was at this time that selenium was used as an effective remedy for other livestock diseases and that it was first linked to vitamin E. Vitamin E could replace or accompany selenium in treating these livestock diseases. New Zealand was the first country to make widespread use of the mineral to prevent deficiency problems in domestic animals. This occurred in 1967 and was due to the fact that New Zealand is one of the areas in the world with the lowest levels of soil selenium. In the same year, Finnish vets used selenium to treat muscle diseases in domestic animals, and in 1969 veterinary authorities authorized the addition of selenium in animal feeds. Also, since 1984 selenium is added to all artificial fertilizers to increase the selenium intake of agricultural products and hence increase the intake of the human population.

Selenium and health

In the 1970s researchers discovered that selenium could prevent mutations, which are unusual changes in genetic material that may trigger disease. Such mutations may be entirely harmless or they may prevent basic processes required for life, and these changes may be passed on to the next generation. Then, in 1973, the enzyme glutathione peroxidase was found. Glutathione peroxidase contains four atoms of selenium in its structure, and it acts against oxygen-free radicals, hydrogen peroxides and fatty acid peroxides, preventing damage to the cell. This finding proved that selenium was very important in preventing animal diseases. Even today, some health practitioners are sceptical about the importance and benefits that selenium can bring in preventing disease. The first serious cases of selenium deficiency in humans arose in the late 1970s in the province of Keshan in China. People there had developed a disease of the heart, similar to 'mulberry heart' of cattle, in which the heart muscle degenerated with a subsequent loss of power to pump blood around the body. It arose mainly in young women and children in an area with possibly the lowest selenium levels in the world. Without selenium supplementation the disease was fatal. A similar disease affecting the cartilage in the joints, called Kaschin-Beck disease, was found in Russia and China, which again could be prevented and treated with selenium supplements.

Requirements for selenium

The human requirements for selenium are not yet known but an intake of 50–200μg is said to be sufficient. However, a value of 70μg for men and 50μg for women is considered enough to keep the balance of selenium absorbed and excreted in step. This level does not consider the aspect of preventing disease. These levels have been difficult to attain in many areas. Northern Europe has very low selenium levels in the soils and rock. This is because the selenium-rich layers of earth were moved southwards, and the soil left contains little of this micronutrient. This problem has been worsened by the effects of acid rain, pollution and the exhaustion of the soil nutrients, and the excessive use of synthetic fertilizers. As mentioned before, this problem has been partially eradicated by supplementing fertilizers and animal foodstuff with selenium. The lack of the mineral is a particular problem in Scandinavia, where foodstuffs are very low in selenium. The mean daily intake of selenium is 45μg in Denmark and Sweden, 50–70μg in Norway and 90–100μg in Finland, because of the supplements described above. To compare, the Keshan province had a daily intake of less than 10μg per day. This reduced mineral intake shows up in the blood selenium levels. Danes, Swedes, New Zealanders and Egyptians have the lowest recorded levels of selenium in their blood. People in Finland have seen a rise in selenium blood serum from 75μgl^{-1} to 100μgl^{-1}, but some people still have selenium serum levels below 85μgl^{-1}, which appears to be the critical level below which there is an increased risk of cardiovascular disease and cancer. Whole blood selenium values of between 200 and 350μgl^{-1} exist because of selenium supplements and confer several protective effects on the body by inhibiting lipid peroxidation and other beneficial effects.

Selenium occurs in an organic form in food, and as both an organic and inorganic form in food supplements. The two types of selenium are absorbed in different ways, with organic selenium being almost totally absorbed (85–95 per cent) but inorganic selenium differing in absorption from 40 to 70 per cent, depending on the type of preparation. Inorganic selenium is lost in the urine when the human body reaches saturation point. Organic selenium is stored in the tissues. In humans there is about 100μgl^{-1}, with 60 per cent of that in the red blood cells while 40 per cent is found in the blood serum. The blood moves the mineral round the tissues and there a proportion of the selenium is bound to the glutathione peroxidase enzyme, while the rest of the mineral is bound to haemoglobin and other proteins. Almost half the total 10–15mg of selenium found in the body is stored in the liver. The activity of glutathione peroxidase is correlated to the levels of selenium in the blood until the enzyme activity reaches an optimal level.

Groups at risk of selenium deficiency

Several groups of the population are liable to a reduced intake of selenium. Young people living away from home may not get a balanced diet because of inadequate funds, lack of time for shopping, lack of proper storage facilities or because of a lack of cooking equipment. Studies in Finland have determined that students get less than half of the average daily intake of selenium. This group may also have the lowest blood selenium levels. Vegetarians' intake of selenium may be as low as $10\mu gl^{-1}$ as grains, plants and vegetables are very low in selenium. The elderly may have inadequate selenium intake as they perhaps cannot afford meat or fish, which contain good amounts of the mineral. Other problems may derive from dental problems as elderly people may struggle to chew or eat meat and fish. Smokers have a greater demand for the antioxidant properties of selenium as smoking and drinking alcohol increase the formation of free radicals. Thus smokers require more of the mineral and almost always have lower blood selenium levels than nonsmokers. People suffering from chronic illnesses, including gastrointestinal diseases such as malabsorption or gluten allergy, may be deficient in selenium. Drugs or diseases that cause loss of appetite, diarrhoea, frequent vomiting and unvaried diets can also result in insufficient selenium. Lower blood selenium levels are seen in most cancer patients as well as in heart disease patients. People with arthritis who are treated using cortisone may lack enough selenium. Pregnant women may become deficient in selenium during pregnancy as the foetus takes part of the mother's selenium reserves for use in its body. While breast-feeding, the mother loses selenium as it is passed to her offspring. This loss can not normally be resolved by a change of diet, and selenium supplements are required to keep up with the mineral losses each day.

The action of selenium in the body

Selenium has a number of different tasks in the human body. As mentioned before, selenium is an antioxidant that prevents peroxidation of lipids in the cells. This halts cell damage and slows the pathological ageing process. Glutathione peroxidase breaks down harmful fatty acid peroxide and hydrogen peroxide. This protective action is complemented by vitamin E and helps in the destruction of these free radicals. Enzymes like superoxide dimutase and catalase also take part in the defence system against free radicals.

Selenium boosts the effectiveness of the immune system by improving the operations of the T-lymphocytes and the macrophages, which scavenge the blood for foreign material. The T-lymphocytes are set to recognize bacteria, virus and cancer cells so they can manufacture antibodies against the invading cells faster. A subset of the T-lymphocytes, called killer T-cells, can eliminate cancer cells. The role of the macrophages is to ingest and destroy human cells that have become infected by viruses or bacteria, and this exposed the pathogen to the antibodies and B-cells. It also stops the pathogen replicating further.

Selenium is linked to the prostaglandins, but by which mechanism is yet unknown. There are 'good' and 'bad' prostaglandins, but selenium appears to raise the production levels of the 'good' prostaglandin chemicals (PGE1 and PGE3). These hormone-like unsaturated fatty acids have a substantial regulatory effect on the coagulation of the blood and also influence the occurrence of arteriosclerosis and the clotting of blood platelets. Hence, these substances have a role in preventing thromboses. Low levels of selenium in the blood serum (less than $85\mu gl^{-1}$) may elevate the chances of having a low level of the HDL-cholesterol, which is the 'good' form, and may increase the risk of a blood clot forming. Low levels of selenium may show as abnormalities on an electrocardiogram and specify heart problems. A low selenium intake seems to be a factor in cases of myocardial infarction and arteriosclerosis.

This mineral has been found to inhibit the toxic effects of heavy metals such as mercury, cadmium, lead and arsenic. The way that selenium protects the body's cells from damage is still to be uncovered. Selenium also protects cells against other harmful substances, like cytotoxic drugs given during chemotherapy. Work has shown that when selenium is given with adriamycin, the adverse side effects are reduced. Adriamycin is a medicine used to treat ovarian cancer, and it encourages the formation of free radicals and is very harmful to the heart and liver. The severity of the action of this drug is tempered by the protective action of selenium.

Selenium and cancer

Experiments on animals have told us that insufficient selenium in our bodies increases the risk of developing cancer. Food supplements of 1–5 parts per million of selenium can repress skin cancer, breast cancer, leukaemia, sarcomas, liver cancer and cancer of the large intestines. Selenium supplements can prevent many cancers forming in animals. This mineral can inhibit the transfer of Bittner's milk virus from the mother to the foetus. This disease occurs in rats, and it and similar viruses are carcinogenic and can be stopped by selenium. These anti-cancer properties can be reinforced by vitamins A and E, when they increase the success rate against cancer in animals from 50 per cent to 90 per cent.

In humans there is a proven link between insufficient selenium and cancer. People with low blood levels of this mineral show a higher occurrence of cancer. This was first detected in the United States in the 1960s because of diet differences from state to state. Many studies have reported that cancer patients with diseases affecting the kidneys, bladder, breast, ovaries, prostate, blood, skin and the rectum show selenium levels in blood and tissue that are 30 per cent lower than those in a healthy control group. One problem with this is that a sick person will not eat the same food or have as good an appetite as a healthy person, so you cannot assume that low selenium status causes cancer. To get over this problem, investigations of healthy people were followed up over many years. These studies showed that the people who developed cancer had low selenium values for years before the disease was detected. Lack of vitamin E and selenium increased the chances of getting cancer by a factor of ten, said one of the recent major studies in Finland. If lack of selenium is associated with deficiencies of other antioxidant vitamins and minerals, e.g. beta-carotene, vitamin A, vitamin E, copper, zinc, manganese, then the probability of getting cancer is heightened further. Selenium appears to fend off cancer in four ways:

1. Selenium protects the cells from damage caused by oxygen-free radicals. These compounds are highly reactive and form peroxides, which accelerate the promotion phase of cancer. This is the stage where precancerous cells are formed.
2. Selenium lowers the mutagenic power of carcinogenic chemicals. This means that the chemicals, viruses and radiation cause less damage to the genetic material in cells.
3. Selenium does not allow carcinogenic viruses to reproduce.
4. Selenium curbs the division of cancer cells and halts them spreading through the tissues.

Despite the myriad activities of selenium, it must not be forgotten that there are many interacting factors that trigger cancers to develop. Selenium has been used since 1911 as a treatment for cancer, boosting antioxidant levels and reinforcing the immune defence. This uses higher doses than are used in preventing disorders, when 200–300μg is the dosage used.

The heart and selenium

Insufficient selenium in cattle causes a disease called 'mulberry heart'. The heart muscle degenerates, and it is left weakened and is unable to pump blood around the body effectively. A similar disease of humans that first arose in the Keshan province in China has been discussed earlier. A few cases of a similar disease appeared, but these were in very ill people who were being drip-fed and who lacked selenium in the parenteral nutrition they were given.

A study carried out in Finland in 1982 showed that when serum levels of selenium were less than 45μgl^{-1}, the chances of contracting heart disease were elevated by a factor between 2 and 7. This work determined that serum levels of under 85μgl^{-1} were associated with the risk factors leading to coronary heart disease, e.g. increased aggregation of platelets, low HDL-cholesterol, and changes in the electrocardiogram pattern during exercise. People with acute myocardial infarction are frequently lacking in selenium and vitamin B$_6$. Other antioxidant vitamins such as A, C and E and the mineral zinc can protect the heart from ischaemia and reperfusion injury. Best results are obtained from a mixture of water-soluble and fat-soluble antioxidants. A British investigation done in the late 1980s found that people with heart infarction and arteriosclerosis have quantities of lipid peroxides (rancid fat) in their blood and that this may be the cause of the problem. This theory is backed up by animal experiments. The size of myocardial infarction can be reduced by antioxidants.

Using selenium for chronic diseases

Selenium may be linked with preventing some children's neurological diseases. Therapy with a range of antioxidants has helped children with Becker's muscular dystrophy and Duchennes muscular dystrophy. These are similar diseases that cause chronic muscle degeneration. Becker's occurs between the ages of eight and twenty, while Duchennes appears between the ages of three and five. Duchennes affects the muscles of the legs and pelvis, in particular, producing a waddling gait, inward curvature of the spine and contracture of joints. Fatty deposits may form in the calves and harden the muscle, and antioxidants may help to limit this deposition.

Selenium deficiency may be connected to the lipid peroxidation that occurs in multiple sclerosis. This is a progressive disease in which the nerve fibres lose their protective sheath of myelin, a fatty substance. Myelin allows fast movement of nerve impulses along the fibre, and without the myelin sheath, transfer of nerve impulses to the muscles is vastly impaired or impossible. Loss of myelin may be because of the action of free radicals oxidizing the fatty deposits, and hence antioxidants such as selenium can help stop the loss of myelin.

Since any inflammation response triggers the formation of lipid peroxides and free radicals, selenium and other antioxidants should ease rheumatic pains, stiffness in the joints and arthritic complaints. In some cases, supplementation with selenium has helped in the neurological disease myasthenia gravis. Selenium antioxidants and essential fatty acids can help various allergies, such as asthma, hay fever and eczema. Antioxidants and selenium can benefit injuries to nerves and blood vessels in diabetes, as they are damaged by lipid peroxidation. The use of selenium as a prophylatic drug to prevent diabetic eye conditions has progressed well. Recently, selenium deficiency has been detected in a number of patients suffering from Aids, and supplements of selenium are being tested to see if they have any beneficial impact.

Preparations of selenium

Organic preparations of selenium are best absorbed by the body, but the degree to which the body can use it varies, partly because of differences between the different selenium products on the market. The best combination of antioxidants contains selenium, zinc, and vitamins A, B_6, C and E. This contains selenium in the form of L-selenomethionine, which is a form of organic selenium. Inorganic selenium is not as effective in the body, and to have the same effect as organic selenium a much larger dose is needed.

The effectiveness of organic selenium has been shown in tests of breast-feeding mothers, when it was found that organic selenium is absorbed into the mother's body well and then secreted in the breast milk in good levels. The inorganic selenium had much poorer absorption into the mother's body and was not detected in the breast milk at all. So the method of selenium supplementation and the quality of the products are important to gain maximum benefits in this case.

Selenium is possibly the most important trace mineral in our diet. It has such a wide range of protective mechanisms and interacts with many other vitamins and minerals. Continuing research will expand our knowledge about the actions and behaviour of selenium in the human body.

silicon

chemical symbol: Si

Silicon is found in the same group of the periodic table as carbon and has similar chemical properties. This mineral has only been recognized as essential for humans recently, and little is known about its uptake, metabolism and function in our bodies. Silicon occurs in nature mainly as silicon dioxide and as silicate salts. Much of the silicon in our diet comes from milk and vegetables. The mineral is absorbed from the intestines and transported in the blood to the muscles, bones, sinews, nails, cartilage and the brain. Quite large amounts of silicon are contained in the lymph glands. Much of the silicon taken into the human body is excreted in the urine. As yet, the level of silicon required by the human body is unknown, and there are no official RDAs. The average human contains around 7g of the mineral, which is more than for iron or copper, and this suggests that the daily requirement is approximately 20–30mg. Whether or not silicon is deficient in our diets is difficult to decide as we do not know what the optimal levels of silicon are, and it is as yet hard to tell how to measure the levels of silicon in the blood. There is no known deficiency disease linked to silicon.

Like selenium, the organic forms of silicon seem to be absorbed and utilized far more effectively by the body than inorganic silicon. Silicon seems to have the ability to stimulate the osteoblast cells, which make bone. It is also important in making the starting material for the connective tissues. Large concentrations of silicon are found in the osteoblasts and are vital in the activity of these cells. The mineral helps to form the proteins collagen and elastin, which allow connective tissues to contract and become elastic. Silicon has become popular in strengthening hair and nail growth, but these beneficial effects have not been backed by controlled studies. Investigations have proved the benefits silicon brings in encouraging bone formation, and supplements of silicon, fluorine and boron have been recommended to aid healing after a fractured bone. People fitted with a replacement hip joint as a result of fracture or osteoarthritis can benefit from supplements of silicon and boron, which will help new bone mass grow around the new joint and hold it in position. This is especially valuable in elderly people, whose bone growth is slower than in young people. There is a possibility that silicon may be good in preventing and treating osteoporosis. Research is needed to determine how calcium, magnesium, silicon and boron work together to allow bone formation.

Silicon may be linked to the development of arteriosclerosis, as the levels of silicon in the artery walls fall with age, and with the start of arteriosclerosis. This lowering of silicon values may cause arteriosclerosis or it may be an effect of the disease. Silicon would appear to help inflammatory reactions as well. The experience of some nutritional doctors shows that supplements of silicon may help strengthen skin, hair and nails and can treat inflammatory skin complaints such as atopic eczema.

zinc

chemical symbol: Zn

Zinc is a metallic element that is very important for good health. It is involved in many processes in the body and controls the functioning of many enzymes. The average human adult contains 2–4g of zinc, of which 78 per cent is held in the bones, muscles and the skin. These tissues store the mineral, and if a deficiency of the mineral arises then the zinc is released. Hence, we require a daily intake of zinc in our diet.

The RDA for zinc is 15mg for adults, but most people do not get this level in their diet. Groups particularly at risk of insufficient zinc are growing children, the elderly, pregnant women, vegetarians and people suffering from chronic illnesses or allergies. During pregnancy and breast-feeding, the levels of zinc required rise by 50 to 75 per cent to 23–27mg daily. Zinc is found in liver, red meat, egg yolk, whole-grain flour, seafood (especially oysters), dairy produce, vegetables, and cereals and their products. The percentage of zinc absorbed in the body is variable, and in a mixed diet of meat and vegetables roughly 15–40 per cent of the zinc intake is absorbed. Zinc in vegetables is not absorbed as well, so vegetarians are at a particular risk of deficiency, and supplementation may be sensible. The best form of zinc, which is absorbed well, is organic zinc, normally as gluconate or aspartate salts. Care should be taken with zinc supplements as zinc competes with copper, and higher levels of zinc intake can reduce the absorption of copper. Any zinc supplement of more than 30mg daily taken to augment the dietary intake should be combined with a small supplement of copper to prevent any problems arising. Zinc is taken in via the intestines and is removed from the body with secretions from the gall bladder and pancreas and with the excreted material. Loss of zinc increases because of diabetes, dialysis treatment, diuretic medicine, some anti-arthritis medicines and excessive sweat production. Tissue damage caused by kidney diseases, flaking skin diseases or burns also cause more zinc to be lost from the body.

Zinc has a multitude of roles in the body. It forms part of the active site of around 200 enzymes, including carbonic anhydrases and dehydrogenases involved in energy metabolism. These enzymes work to form bone tissue, to heal wounds and sores, to produce protein and to regulate the carbohydrate metabolism. Other enzymes are involved in regulating the synthesis of ribosomes and ribonucleic acids. Deficiency of zinc inhibits the growth of children. The mineral forms an essential part of the CuZn superoxide dismutase (SOD) enzyme, which is an antioxidant that neutralizes harmful free radicals. Zinc helps boost the immune system against invading viruses, bacteria, allergens and carcinogens, and inadequate zinc intake lessens our disease resistance. Other of the enzymes activated by zinc is the enzyme that converts retinol to retinal, which is used to form eye pigments. Lack of zinc means the body cannot utilize the vitamin A it receives in the diet and the body is lacking in the antioxidant vitamin A. Zinc also forms part of the enzyme that allows the release of insulin from the pancreas. Zinc is also needed to transform one of the essential fatty acids, linoleic acid, into gamma-linolenic acid, which is required for the production of 'good' prostaglandins.

Zinc deficiency causes problems with the skin, because 20 per cent of the body's reserves are stored in the skin, and this tissue reacts fast to deficiency conditions. Insufficient zinc can also cause slow physical, mental and sexual development. It can affect and reduce the healing of wounds, and it may be important in infertility. Inadequate zinc levels can cause decreased alertness, poor appetite, increased susceptibility to infection and injury, retarded growth and a loss of the sense of smell. Hormonal disturbances, general fatigue and losing the sense of taste can result from too little zinc. This mineral has attracted a great deal of attention lately as lack of zinc appears to be connected with dysfunctions of the brain, such as dyslexia. In a British study, children with the condition had zinc values a third lower than their classmates without the condition. This was followed up by an investigation in Finland, where 18 children with dyslexia were given supplements of 15mg of zinc and 100μg of selenium daily. Analysis showed that prior to the study 13 out of the 18 children had lower zinc concentrations in their blood than normal. After eight months of supplementation, 11 children showed significant improvements and had less difficulty in reading and writing. The schoolteachers reported a substantial improvement was seen in the whole class after only two months of mineral supplementation. Many in the medical profession believe that dyslexia may derive from zinc deficiencies in one of the parents when the child is conceived. Zinc is also thought to be linked with the circumference of the baby's skull. Low zinc levels in the placenta are associated with small skull circumference and related delays in brain development.

Zinc is used as a therapy for several diseases, including acne, heart diseases, stomach ulcers and arthritis, and benefits the healing of skin wounds as it speeds up the healing process. The mineral may be good used before and after operations to aid healing. When taken in combination with vitamins A, B_6, C and E, zinc is very helpful for skin diseases and allergic problems like hay fever. Zinc should be taken by cancer patients as it helps to limit the spread of the tumour, and a dose of 15–30mg per day would be most effective. The mineral is being used to treat an eye disease, called senile degeneration of the macula, which causes impaired sight or blindness in elderly people. The disease is caused or worsened by free radicals, and the zinc forms part of essential enzymes that are needed for correct eye functioning.

Fortunately, zinc is not too toxic, and side effects are unlikely even with considerable overdosing. In doses of more than 30mg per day, when taken for a period of time, it is best to take a copper supplement, both to avoid copper deficiency and to avoid a possible increase in the cholesterol levels in the blood.

Trace Elements

arsenic
chemical symbol: As

Many people will wonder about including this mineral in a list of minerals essential for health. Arsenic has been seen as a poison for many years, and recent medical studies have shown that arsenic may be required, in small quantities, for the correct functioning of the human body. An adult contains about 14mg of arsenic, and it is estimated that the daily requirements are between 0.5 and 4.0mg. Arsenic is stored in all the tissues, especially the hair and nails. Investigations using experimental animals showed that when the dietary intake of arsenic is less than 0.5mg per kilogram of body weight, the animals' growth and fertility are affected and their internal organs are at risk from damage. Arsenic is used in some drugs to try and kill the Trypanosomas parasite, which is found in Africa and Central and South America and which is transmitted to humans by various insects. Poisoning by arsenic can be chronic, with symptoms of nausea, headache, dry and pigmented skin, hair loss and tiredness, or acute, which shows as nausea, diarrhoea, vomiting and sweating, all stemming from inflammation of the stomach lining. Poisoning by arsenic can be counteracted by selenium, and vice versa. Environmental exposure to arsenic, e.g. through mining, can give rise to a specific form of lung cancer. The incidence of this cancer is reduced if the miners have high levels of selenium in their blood.

boron
chemical symbol: B

The element is similar to aluminium, and it is the subject of a lot of medical and scientific studies that show it is an essential trace element. Boron is essential to animals and plants. It is found in tomatoes, pears, prunes, raisins, dates, berries, apples, citrus fruits and avocados. Wine, soya meal, nuts, and honey are also rich in boron. At the moment, there is no RDA for boron, but it has been calculated that 1–2mg of boron per day may meet the human requirement. Most people consume between 1 and 2mg of boron each day, although intakes of only 0.25mg have been seen. The levels of boron in fruit and vegetables depends on the levels of the mineral in the soil. Mauritius and Jamaica have low levels of boron and may not get enough boron in their diet. The levels of the mineral in the blood and tissues are sensitive to the variations in diet from day to day, and vegetarians may benefit from the higher levels of boron in their diets from the vegetables.

The main role of boron in the body is unknown, but it appears to be important in preventing and treating osteoporosis and rheumatoid arthritis. People with rheumatoid arthritis or similar joint diseases have significantly lower levels of boron in their bones, when compared to healthy people. Workers in New Zealand found that a daily supplement of 6–9mg of boron would reverse the symptoms in 80–90 per cent of patients within a few weeks of treatment. Boron was also found to cure arthritis in cattle, dogs and horses. Boron in the form of borax ($Na_2B_4O_7.IOH_2O$) has been used to help arthritis in New Zealand and Australia. Countries like Israel, which has high levels of boron in the soil, have virtually no incidence of arthritis, while Jamaica and Mauritius have low soil boron levels and a high incidence of arthritis.

Studies completed by the United States Department of Agriculture show that a supplement of 3mg of boron reduces the amounts of magnesium, calcium and phosphorus excreted in the urine of post-menopausal women. An additional benefit of this therapy was that oestrogen levels in the blood were increased by 100 per cent after only eight days of treatment. This is of great importance as oestrogen reduces demineralization of bones after the menopause. All this evidence points to the idea that dietary deficiency of boron may be involved in osteoporosis in women after the menopause. It would seem that a supplement of 3mg of boron each day would help both prevent and treat osteoporosis and rheumatoid arthritis. Boron may benefit people with allergic reactions as people who suffer from allergic rashes generally have low levels of boron present in their skin.

lead

chemical symbol: Pb

Lead is a metallic element that some sources believe is required by the body in very small quantities. Lead salts may be applied to wounds, when it helps to stop bleeding, reduces inflammation and provides a protective covering over the wound. Large doses of soluble lead salts irritate the stomach. Lead is well known as a poison, and this chronic poisoning occurs most often because of exposure in the workplace. Plumbers, pottery workers, dyers, lead smelters and people cleaning petrol storage tanks are most at risk. Lead may be derived from drinking water contaminated with lead, and the risks are particularly high in areas with soft or peaty water, which are more capable of dissolving lead. Lead can be inhaled as dry dust, absorbed through the skin, or absorbed via the stomach from the diet and water supply. Symptoms of chronic poisoning can start with muscular weakness, constipation, pale skin and colic. The formation of a blue line marking the gums is characteristic of lead poisoning along with anaemia, anorexia and damage to the nervous system causing muscle tremors and paralysis. Lead also causes damage to the kidney function, blindness (temporary or permanent) because of nerve damage, convulsions and death if treatment cannot halt the damage and exposure continues. Acute poisoning is similar, causing abdominal pains, diarrhoea, vomiting and possibly developing into convulsions and paralysis. Treatment is with a chelating agent, which removes the lead from the circulation, and it is eliminated from the body. Evidence varies as to whether lead is important in human health, but its deleterious effects are common knowledge.

nickel

chemical symbol: Ni

This element is a metal, and it is essential for the human body's requirements. Nickel is found in vegetables, explaining why vegetarians tend to have a higher intake of it than people with a mixed meat and vegetable diet. There is no RDA established for nickel, but daily intakes vary from 130 to 400μg. It is poorly absorbed in the intestines, with only 10 per cent absorbed, and this does not increase as intake increases. The excess nickel is eliminated from the body in the faeces, with smaller amounts lost through sweating and in the urine. The normal serum blood levels of nickel are around 1.5–5.0μgl^{-1}. Much of the evidence for nickel being an essential trace element comes from animal experiments, where nickel deficiency leads to a range of complaints. Rats and pigs have reduced growth and lowered fertility when nickel is lacking, and hens show changes to the blood, liver and skin. There are no recognized deficiency diseases for nickel in humans, but it has been discovered that levels in the blood increase when the heart is lacking in oxygen (ischaemia). The nickel in the blood is not released from the heart muscle, and this change is not yet fully understood. It does allow examination of blood nickel values to identify ischaemic heart disease and to determine the level of damage after a heart attack.

Recent studies from Denmark have shown that high blood levels of nickel may be linked to arthritis. Nickel is contained in drinking water as it is released from the metal pipes. This can be a particular occurrence in water that has been left standing in pipes all night, and it can be exceedingly high in the mineral. It is advisable to let water run for a time to reduce the level of nickel in it. Nickel in the diet can cause allergic eczema and in wristwatches or jewellery it can cause an allergic contact dermatitis. Some people even have an allergic reaction to the nickel in coins.

There are no health reasons for using nickel to prevent or treat illness, and nickel carbonyl compounds used in industry are known to be carcinogenic.

tin

chemical symbol: Sn

This is a metal that is vital for proper functioning of the human body. In animal experiments, it was found that rats need 1–2mg of tin per kilogram of body weight so normal growth and development can occur. The level of requirement by humans has not been determined, and there is no RDA set. Fresh food normally contains 1mg of tin in every kilogram of food, while the level of tin in tinned or deep-frozen food is generally 2mg per kilogram of foodstuff. Thus the tin intake varies depending on the amount of frozen or tinned food consumed, from 0.2 to 17mg per day. In the United States, 15 per cent of total food eaten is from tins so they probably have the largest consumption of the mineral. Like selenium and chromium, inorganic salts of tin are absorbed to a much lower extent than organic tin. Both types of tin are excreted differently, with organic tin being lost along with the faeces and inorganic tin with the urine.

The main role of tin is to contribute to the absorption of several other minerals and trace elements. It inhibits the absorption of zinc and copper into some tissues and limits their elimination from the body. In some cases, it can increase the removal of zinc with the urine. Tin does not appear to affect the excretion of manganese, iron or magnesium. Tin does play an important role in the metabolism of bone tissue, possibly in conjunction with vitamin D. Experiments with animals have shown that tin has differing effects on the immune system. Some strengthen the immune system and others may weaken it. It is possible that the growth of cancerous tissue may be halted to some degree by supplementation of the diet with tin. This response may occur through the action of the immune system or the mineral may act on the cells directly. Tin is only slightly toxic, but there is too little evidence to back the use of tin as a treatment for disease. The actions of tin on the immune system and on cancer may become more valuable in the future.

tungsten

chemical symbol: W

This metal normally occurs in nature in compounds of iron. Tungsten is a component of most mixed diets, but it has not been determined whether or not this mineral is an essential trace element. There is currently little information about average daily intakes, and no RDA is established. Tungsten from the diet is stored in the liver, bones and kidneys.

Tungsten has a mutual relationship with other trace elements, especially copper and molybdenum. Absorption of molybdenum from the intestines can be obstructed by tungsten, and it modifies the activity of the enzyme xanthine oxidase, which requires molybdenum to function effectively.

Tungsten itself is not too toxic, but some forms, e.g. tungsten carbide, are liable to cause lung damage. There are no current uses for tungsten in either preventing or treating disease.

vanadium

chemical symbol: V

This metal is recognized as an essential trace element, but unfortunately relatively little is known about it. Vanadium is found in some plants and vegetables, particularly radishes and dill, and only 1 per cent of this mineral from our diet is absorbed into the body, with the rest being removed via the urine. There are no set requirements for vanadium, but we are estimated to need between 1 and 4mg daily. The amount of vanadium present in the average diet is also unknown. The vanadium that is taken into the body is metabolized by a route that we do not know, but most tissues contain vanadium but in quantities that have not yet been worked out. Blood serum levels of vanadium are less than $10\mu gl^{-1}$.

Most of the information about vanadium relates to work completed on animals. Research in 1971 found that rats that had been lacking in vanadium for a long period of time gained approximately 40 per cent of their body weight when they were fed vanadium supplements of sodium orthovanadate. Deficiency in vanadium led to retarded development of chickens and, unexpectedly, to lowered cholesterol levels. These observations cannot be directly transferred to humans. Studies have shown that vanadium can curb the development of spontaneous tumours in animals and may lessen the carcinogenic properties of some chemicals. Conflicting reports on the action of vanadium salts are known, and some studies show that these salts can destroy cancer cells. It is to be hoped that our knowledge about this element and its importance in humans will increase in the future.

Other Minerals

aluminium

chemical symbol: Al

There is considerable debate as to whether aluminium has any benefits to human health. The human requirements for the mineral are not known, but the amount of aluminium in the diet varies from 7mg in Finland, 80mg in Norway to 100mg in the United States. The higher two values take into account aluminium that enters food from the surface of aluminium cooking pots, other kitchen utensils and disposable juice cartons coated with aluminium. It also enters our bodies from environmental pollution in the air, and these unusual sources of the mineral can be quite significant. Aluminium is the third most abundant element in the earth's crust, making up 8 per cent of it. Aluminium is released from the soil by the action of acid rain lowering the pH, and the mineral then enters the ground water and may be taken into supplies of drinking water. Concentrations of aluminium in drinking water in Norway and the United Kingdom seem to correlate to the prevalence of Alzheimer's disease. This possibility is currently being researched further, and more information as to the mechanism of the link is awaited, but it has been proposed that the disease results from the deposition of aluminium in the brain cells, which would impair their functioning.

Aluminium forms part of our diet as instant coffee, table salt, dried milk, some food additives and in tea bags. The mineral is also a component of many stomach medicines, including anti-acid tablets, that can increase the levels of aluminium excreted in the urine by 800 per cent and the excretion of zinc by 125 per cent. Aluminium hydroxide in stomach medicines also binds to phosphates and means they cannot be taken up by the body. This can lead to inadequate levels of phosphorus in the body. Several vaccines for diseases also contain aluminium.

Aluminium is an extremely reactive chemical, and it is inclined to bind to other substances. Since aluminium ions (Al^{3+}) are similar to iron (Fe^{3+}), aluminium can change places with iron in proteins such as ferritin (see iron in Microminerals) and so enter the cells. When in the body, aluminium causes demineralization of the bones, changes the metabolism of calcium and allows cross-linkages to form in collagen. The mineral also brings about zinc loss, and this may play a part in the development of dementia. Dyslexic people often have high levels of

311

aluminium and low levels of zinc in the body. When zinc is lacking, aluminium can bind to proteins that carry zinc, and supplementation with zinc is necessary to reverse the deficiency, correct the protein structures and restore normal function to many enzyme complexes.

Patients who are drip-fed or who need dialysis treatment absorb much more aluminium than normal people, and this can cause damage to bones and brain damage. This is why dialysis fluids are normally purified and the aluminium removed because aluminium poisoning can be fatal.

silver

chemical symbol: Ag

This element is not required by the human body for any metabolic processes. It is used in medicine as an antiseptic and astringent, and has been used against warts and to stop nosebleeds. In studies of experimental animals, silver given in the diet was only slightly absorbed into the body (10 per cent of the total). The mineral is transported to the liver and stored there. It is not known if the same process happens in humans.

Silver has mutual effects with the minerals copper and selenium and with vitamin E. This means that silver can protect an organism against overdoses and poisoning by these substances, and vice versa. Chronic silver poisoning shows as a permanent blue colouring of the connective membrane in the eye. Poisoning by silver salts, such as silver nitrate, causes discolouring of the lips, abdominal pains, dizziness, vomiting and convulsions.

gold

chemical symbol: Au

Gold is similar to silver in that it is not an essential mineral for humans. It is used to treat some diseases. Gold was first used as a medicine by Jacques Forestier, a Frenchman, about in the middle of the 20th century. He thought that rheumatoid arthritis might be a form of tuberculosis and, as such a serious illness, it would have to be treated with the most expensive medicines. Gold salts are absorbed from the gastrointestinal tract very poorly and have mainly been replaced by chelate gold preparations, which enter the blood and tissues easily. This mineral has also been administered as intramuscular injections, and this produces high concentrations of gold in the tissues. Approximately 5 per cent of the gold administered is excreted after a day, and 85 per cent of the dose is still present after one week. Gold is still being eliminated with the urine as long as one year after injection.

The main use of gold is as treatment for rheumatoid arthritis, as it appears to subdue the inflammatory response in the joints. How this occurs is not entirely understood, but a Japanese study proposed that gold functioned as an antioxidant. This belief may be correct as supplementation with the antioxidants selenium and zinc does not conflict with the use of gold as a therapy. Metallic gold is used by dentists for filling teeth, but has also been utilized in surgery and to treat asthma and skin diseases. Gold is not an essential mineral so it can cause side effects in some patients, with itching, serious kidney damage and rashes. The level of kidney damage is not linked to the dose given but to the degree of sensitivity of the patient to gold treatment. Unfortunately, gold can cause serious toxicity in 10 per cent of patients treated for rheumatoid arthritis and has some toxic reaction in between 25 per cent and 50 per cent of them.

Essential Fatty Acids

Essential fatty acids (EFA) were previously called the F vitamins. They are a group of polyunsaturated fatty acids that are vital for the proper functioning, growth and maintenance of the body. Our requirements of these substances are met entirely through our diet, and deficiencies can occur in some circumstances. We are recommended that at least 10–15 per cent of our intake of calories should come from essential fatty acids. The first EFA was discovered in 1929, and we now know of 12 essential fatty acids, but only linoleic and linolenic acids are required in the diet as the body can transform them into all the other EFAs.

The main essential fatty acids are:

—linoleic acid: found in seed oils of blackcurrants, sunflowers, maize, peanuts, borage and evening primrose.

—gamma-linolenic acid (GLA): found in the seeds of borage, evening primrose and blackcurrants and also in breast milk.

—dihomo-gamma-linolenic acid (DHGLA): contained in offal and breast milk.

—alpha-linolenic acid: found in linseed, soya beans and vegetables.

—arachidonic acid: contained in dairy products, meat, marine algae and prawns.

—eicosapentaenoic acid (EPA): found in marine algae, fish liver oil and fatty fish, e.g. salmon, herring, mackerel.

—docosahexaenoic acid (DHA): found in fish, fish liver oil and marine algae.

Interest in these chemicals has increased in recent years, and there are many medical studies being carried out to determine if they can prevent or treat diseases successfully. Most of this work is centred on the effect of EFAs on heart disease, failure of the immune system, disorders of the central nervous system, and allergies. The EFAs are important as the cell membranes are all made up of fatty acids, and these membranes are critical for cell functioning so a lack of EFAs can give rise to serious tissue problems. EFAs are also required as precursors of prostaglandins (PG) and leukotrienes, which are hormone-like substances. Leukotrienes are made from arachdonic acid and are important in inflammation and allergic reactions. They can cause swelling and fluid accumulation in tissues and cause a very strong contraction of the respiratory passages (around 1000 times stronger contraction than is caused by histamine). Prostaglandins have a larger role and work in capsule, which reduces both the cost and the number of capsules needed to be taken each day. The initial high dosage required to treat some complaints does not need to be sustained, and the dose can be reduced to the minimum dose and the treatment is still effective. When taking any supplement of essential fatty acids, the body should have sufficient antioxidants to stop the possible rancification of the EFAs.

eicosapentanoic acid (EPA) *and* docosahexanoic acid (DHA)

These essential fatty acids are also known as omega–3 fatty acids or fish oils. Their reputation as beneficial for health has hugely increased in recent years, and several studies have confirmed their worth. The human body can produce EPA and DHA from linoleic acid but not in adequate quantities. In the diet they are found in fish, especially fatty fish like salmon, herring and mackerel, fish oils, marine algae, linseeds, and in meat from marine mammals, such as seals and whales, which are eaten in certain cultures. Interest arose when it was found that Eskimos and Japanese fishermen, both groups who ate a lot of fish, had a very low occurrence of heart disease. This connection was then studied in large controlled tests, and a significant link does occur between high intake of fish (and so EPA and DHA) and vastly reduced levels of heart disease. These studies also showed that the incidence of psoriasis, diabetes, asthma and sclerosis were rarer in the groups with a fish-rich diet.

Heart disease is connected to the amount of food consumed and the way in which our diet is balanced between protein, carbohydrate and fats. Generally, the more fat in the diet the higher the risk of heart disease. The levels of cholesterol in the blood as LDL-cholesterol (and its oxidized form o-LDL) increase the risk of hardening of the coronary arteries, while HDL-cholesterol is the protective form of the substance. The impact of cholesterol levels can build up over the long term, even over decades, against the action of dietary fat levels, which affect the aggregation of blood platelets and blood clot formation directly. The tendency of platelets to gather is increased by saturated fats in the diet, and polyunsaturated fats, especially fish oils, discourage this aggregation.

The actions of EPA and DHA are linked to the production of prostaglandins and leukotrienes. These hormone-like substances act in a localized way in the body and are described in the section on gamma-linolenic acid (GLA) above. Fish oils shift the balance towards prostaglandins, which reduce the risks of blood clot formation. EPA and DHA are transformed into prostaglandins, such as thromboxane A3(TXA3) and prostacyclin (PGE13), which lower the aggregation of platelets in the blood. EPA and DHA also allow the blood cells to pass through the blood capillaries. These capillaries are the smallest blood vessels in the body and are only wide enough to allow red blood cells through in a single stream, approximately 7–10μm in diameter. This is why EPA and DHA can help prevent ischaemic heart disease, as they prevent blood cells sticking in the tiny vessels and causing oxygen deficiency in the heart tissue.

Fish oils have been shown to help chronic conditions such as psoriasis, migraines, arthritis and atopic eczema. This is why most governments and health authorities encourage people to eat fish at least twice a week. Along with that, they advise a reduction in the intake of animal fats, which directly oppose the beneficial effects of fish oils. There are now many products containing fish oil, of varying quality. Capsules of fish oil cannot give rise to the allergic reactions some people have to the protein contained in fish flesh. Fish oils, which contain free fatty acids, have an excellent rate of uptake into the body and would be the most effective preparation currently available.

As with GLA, the polyunsaturated fatty acids EPA and DHA in the diet and supplements are very easily oxidized in the body, so care should be taken to ensure an adequate intake of antioxidants such as selenium and vitamin E so that the benefits to health are not lost.

Vitamin and Mineral RDA Ranges

RDA values (recommended dietary allowance)

Vitamin or mineral	RDA range
A	4–5000 IU retinol; 750–1000μg; 4.5mg beta-carotene
B$_1$	1.0–1.5mg
B$_2$	1.1–3.0mg
B$_3$	18–20mg niacin; 1.08mg tryptophan
B$_5$	5–50mg
B$_6$	1.5–2.2mg
B$_9$	200–400μg
B$_{12}$	1–6μg
C	30mg/60mg
D	400 IU; 2.5–10μg
E	12–30 IU; 10mg
K	either 70–140μg (0.07–0.14mg) or > 1mg
biotin	0.1mg–0.3mg
calcium	500–1000mg
chlorine	no RDA
chromium	50–200μg
cobalt	no RDA
copper	50–2500μg
fluorine	1–4mg
iodine	100–200μg
iron	10–18mg
magnesium	300–450mg
manganese	2.5–3.8mg
molybdenum	100–500μg
phosphorus	800–1000mg
potassium	1–6g
selenium	50–200μg
sodium	2–3g
zinc	15mg
arsenic	0.5–4.0mg safe intake

Counting Calories

boron	1–2mg safe intake
bromine	1.5–2.5mg normal dietary intake
nickel	130–400μg normal dietary intake
tin	0.2–17mg normal dietary intake
vanadium	1–4mg estimated dietary requirement
aluminium	7–100mg normal dietary intake
tungsten	no RDA
lead	no RDA